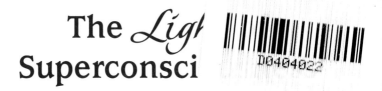

The *Light* of Superconsci

How to Benefit From Emerging Spiritual Trends

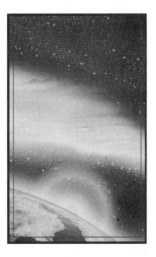

J. Donald Walters
(Swami Kriyananda)

Edited by Devi Novak

Cover and book design by C. A. Starner Schuppe
Photo of J. Donald Walters by Mel Bly
Photo of Devi Novak by Robert Govinda Frutos

Printed in the United States of America

ISBN: 1-56589-748-X

Crystal

Clarity

Crystal Clarity, Publishers
14618 Tyler-Foote Road
Nevada City, CA 95959-8599

Phone: 800-424-1055 or 530-478-7600
Fax: 530-478-7610
E-mail: clarity@crystalclarity.com
Website: www.crystalclarity.com

1 3 5 7 9 8 6 4 2

Library of Congress Cataloging-in-Publication Data
Walters, J. Donald.
    The light of superconsciousness : how to benefit from emerging
spiritual trends / J. Donald Walters ; edited by Devi Novak.
        p. cm.
    Includes bibliographical references.
    ISBN 1-56589-748-X (pbk.)
    1. Spiritual life. 2. Self-realization--Religious aspects.
3. Ananda Cooperative Village--Doctrines. I. Novak, Devi.
II. Title.
BP605.S4W35 1999
299' .93--dc21   99-36570
                                                    CIP

Dedication

This book is dedicated to
The power of love to change our lives—
As I have learned it from
My guru, Paramhansa Yogananda,
My teacher, Swami Kriyananda,
My husband, my son and his family, and
My friends throughout the Ananda Communities.

Preface

"I've come to show you who and what you really are."

—Paramhansa Yogananda

A friend of mine whose life-long love was organic gardening once told me something very intriguing. He said that all life on earth is sustained by the interaction of the uppermost millimeter of soil with air and sunlight. The microorganisms living in the soil are thereby regenerated, making the soil fertile and allowing seeds to germinate into the plants that feed us. Ultimately, of course, life is a divine creation, but the prosaic elements of earth and air serve as the instruments that allow this to happen.

If we look sensitively, we realize that a similar process happens in our soul. All spiritual life is sustained by the subtle interaction between the soil of a receptive mind and the enriching elements of the divine wisdom and compassion of an enlightened teacher. This process cannot occur in the arid earth of our rational mind, but requires the fertile soil of our soul-awareness, or super-consciousness. So, just as with the regeneration of life, this renewal of spirit is ultimately an act of divine grace, but the humble servants of God activate His power for us.

For the past thirty years I've seen this process of spiritual awakening take place in people around the world through the wisdom and compassion of two great souls: the great Indian master, Paramhansa Yogananda, and his direct disciple, Swami Kriyananda. Guru and disciple met in 1948, when a twenty-two-year-old J. Donald

Walters (later known as Swami Kriyananda) read his master's book, *Autobiography of a Yogi,* and took the next bus from New York to Los Angeles to be with him. For the past 50 years, Kriyananda has dedicated his life to spreading Yogananda's teachings through lectures, books, and music, and through the founding of Ananda Village in 1968. Ananda is a spiritual community located outside of Nevada City, California, where hundreds of people live together as they learn and practice these teachings. Today there are four other branch communities located in the United States and one near Assisi, Italy.

I first heard Swami Kriyananda lecture shortly after I came to Ananda in 1969. I was struck by the depth and breadth of his knowledge, by his wonderful humor, but, most of all, by his devotion to his guru, and the intensity of his search for God. His lectures were spontaneous, and, as he told us, not prepared in advance. Yet they reflected a lifetime of spiritual dedication and insight, as well as being keenly responsive to the needs and unspoken questions in the minds of those present. It has been a privilege for me to edit this book, and to share with you the teachings that have changed my life.

This book is composed of ten lectures given over a period of two and a half weeks from January 9th–28th, 1996. The first talk took place at Ananda Village, and the subsequent ones were given during a tour of the Ananda sister communities in Seattle, Washington; Portland, Oregon; and Sacramento and Palo Alto, California. Several of the talks were given at celebrations for Yogananda's birthday, which is on January 5th. I suggest that you read them in the order given, because each talk builds on the ideas and inspiration of the previous ones. I've tried to keep the spontaneous tone of the talks, and where there were questions from the audience, these are included.

The light of superconsciousness—the light of God that shines in each of us—is filled with power, grace, and the deepest love. This light is reflected in the pages you're about to read, and perhaps you'll find it reflected within you as well. For as Yogananda said over and again, "I've come to show you who and what you really are." We *are* the light of superconsciousness, and we are all moving ineluctably toward this divine realization.

Devi Novak
Ananda Village
December 29, 1998

Contents

Preface 4

Introduction 9

1.   The Cycles of Time—Keys to Planetary Evolution 13

2.   Worshipping God as Divine Mother 27

3.   A Tribute to Yogananda 53

4.   Kriya Yoga—The Universal Science 75

5.   Paramhansa Yogananda—The Power of Divine Love 93

6.   Ananda Village—How It Was Started, and Why 114

7.   How to Be a True Disciple 140

8.   A Cosmic Vision of Unity 160

9.   Karma, Free Will, and Realization 176

10. The Light of Superconsciousness—

                The Dawn of a New Age 194

        Glossary 217

        About the Author and the Editor 219

        Other Resources 220

Introduction

Paramhansa Yogananda was one of the first great Indian masters of yoga to make his home in the West. From his arrival in America in 1920 until his death in 1952, he was constantly active and creative in making the teachings of the great seers of past millennia relevant and practical for modern Westerners. His teachings cover a broad range of topics, but there are two aspects that hold particular importance for us now: his techniques for achieving superconsciousness, or Self-realization, and his insights into the future of the human race.

What Is Superconsciousness?

Paramhansa Yogananda used the term "superconsciousness" to refer to that level of awareness that is achieved when the individual merges with Infinite consciousness. From this state we feel unity with all creation; we're able to grasp the subtlest truths of the universe; and we can tap into an unlimited stream of energy and creative solutions in our life.

Yogananda describes his first experience of this state of superconsciousness in his *Autobiography of a Yogi*: "An oceanic joy broke upon calm endless shores of my soul. The Spirit of God, I realized, is exhaustless Bliss; His body is countless tissues of light. A swelling glory within me began to envelop towns, continents, the earth, solar and stellar systems, tenuous nebulae, and floating universes. The entire cosmos, gently luminous, like a city seen afar at night, glimmered within the infinitude of my being."

This superconscious level of perception is something attainable by everyone. Through the practical techniques of yoga and meditation that Yogananda brought to the West, he has made high states of spiritual development accessible to all who sincerely seek them.

Why Are These Teachings so Important Now?

Although most of us are aware that profound changes are happening around us today, it's hard to fit them together into a meaningful picture. We can see many outward manifestations—the advances in communication and in storing information, the breakthroughs in science and physics, the great popularity of alternative healing, and a renewed interest in spirituality of all kinds. It's like watching a new building going up—we can see that something is being created, but we can't tell what it will look like when it's finished.

As we move into a new millennium, we need to turn to those who have brought this light of superconsciousness into the world. Their mission is to usher in a new dawn of spiritual awareness for our planet. Yogananda offers us deep insight into *why* the "new age" is happening and what it will look like. He foresaw neither the end of the world, as some doomsday prophets expound, or a golden age, as other self-styled psychics promise. Rather he drew from ancient yogic traditions, and explained that we are moving into an "Age of Energy." This will be a time of the breaking down of old religious, social, and political forms, of accelerated personal growth, and increased global unity.

How to Live in the Age of Energy

The themes presented in this book show us how to live in this new age of energy and how to benefit from the trends that will be emerging in it. The new expressions of religion will be non-dogmatic and non-sectarian.

They will lead to a uniting of science and religion as people realize that there are practical tools and techniques for spiritual growth. The divisions between men and women will be broken down as people realize the importance of the feminine energy in both religion and daily life. Devotion and the energy of the heart will be understood as essential for human happiness. The need for spiritual training and discipleship will be understood, and the guru-disciple relationship will find true appreciation.

Social patterns will change from people living in huge urban cities to small rural cooperative communities where new ideas and creative expression can flourish. We will begin to understand how to break old patterns of action and thought, how to free ourselves from the limitations of karmic compulsions, and to realize that as beings of energy—not matter—we do have free will.

And we will realize our own potential to draw energy from the world around us. This energy is unlimited, and we can use it for greater mental clarity, greater health and well-being, greater creativity and accomplishment, and ultimately for realization of our oneness with God.

This is what *The Light of Superconsciousness* is all about. It is the teachings of Paramhansa Yogananda as presented by his direct disciple, Swami Kriyananda. Sometimes Kriyananda refers to his guru as "Yogananda," sometimes as "Master," which alludes to his state of complete self-mastery. Through the power of his unity with God, Yogananda was able to show a new vision of reality to all who are seeking.

This book offers us a blueprint for the future which is so essential in the present time of transition. Our civilization has a tremendous potential to see the world in a new way—not as form and matter, but as energy and light; not as divisions and separate political states, but as a unified world family. Technology is paving the way for us, but without a change in our consciousness, the incredible potential for human growth that lies before us will not be achieved. For those who recognize what this challenge means, we need to dedicate ourselves to supporting the emerging spiritual trends and to making this new dawn of superconscious a reality on our planet.

Chapter One

![decorative symbol]

The Cycles of Time—Keys to Planetary Evolution

"The discoveries that lie ahead of us are enormous, but all of it will be based on, one way or another, an awareness of energy as the underlying reality."

At one time or another most of us cast a baleful eye at the events of history and ask ourselves, "What does all this mean? Is it all just a succession of battles and conquests, or is there some grand scheme to it all?" Many ancient cultures asked these same questions, and arrived at the conclusion that mankind must move through different ages or stages of development. The Egyptians called them the Ages of Men, of Heroes, of Demi-Gods, and of the Gods. The Greeks described them as the Iron Age, the Bronze Age, the Silver Age, and the Golden Age. This is all very interesting, but it always seems to be based on mythology rather than on any historical or scientific fact. How does this help us to understand both the pageant of history, and where we are right now?

According to the ancient teachings of India, there are four ages, or *yuga*s, that move in a continuous cycle from highest to lowest and back to the highest. Many Indian writers have tried to make a case for the fact that once you are at the lowest age, there's a sudden leap back to the highest. But that's not the way nature does anything; you don't go from midnight to noon. Everything in nature is cyclical and gradual, and the progression of the ages reflects this.

The explanation the ancient seers give for this progression is that our sun has a dual, and the two revolve around each other within our galaxy. In this revolution they move in a great elliptical orbit toward, then away from, a tremendous vortex of energy which lies at the center of our galaxy. The yugas represent the progression from the time when our sun and solar system are the farthest from the center of the galaxy to the time when we're the closest.

In Sri Yukteswar's book, *The Holy Science,* which he wrote in 1894, he discusses these ideas—the cycle of the yugas, our solar dual, and the great galactic center. At the time he wrote this, science had no idea about such things—people didn't even know back then that there were other galaxies, but thought that our galaxy was the whole of the universe. It wasn't until fairly recently, in 1918, that scientists discovered that what they thought of as a gaseous nebula around Andromeda was actually a whole galactic system. Then they discovered one or two more. I remember that when I was a schoolboy in the 1930s, people were astounded to realize that there were actually as many as three other galaxies apart from our own. Now, of course, they know that there are at least a hundred billion galaxies, but this knowledge is very recent.

A few years ago astronomers also began talking about the possible existence of a solar dual, or dark star. When Sri Yukteswar talked of our moving toward the center of the galaxy, scientists didn't know it existed. Now, in fact, they say we are moving toward that center, and that a tremendous radiation of energy is coming from it. Their instruments can't measure spiritual energy, but they can measure physical energy, and it's coming out in huge amounts from the center of the galaxy.

Sri Yukteswar explained that rays of spiritual energy pour out from this great central sun, and as we come closer to it, more energy floods our planet. Because of this increased energy, people's consciousness becomes more aware. Sri Yukteswar is the first person, to my knowledge, to give an explanation for a teaching that was known back in ancient times, but that we've lost touch with and couldn't explain anymore. In fact, it's because we're moving into an age of greater enlightenment that we can understand it at all.

When our solar system, revolving around its dual, moves away from that center of energy, the result is that human consciousness becomes duller, not able to understand things as well. It reached its farthest point from the galactic center in roughly 500 AD, which was the heart of the Dark Ages. Now it's moving toward the center again, and human consciousness, getting more energy, is able to understand things better. We're beginning to recognize, for example, that matter is not essentially solid, but that it's really energy.

We can observe with our own eyes that the basic difference between people of genius and people of mental dullness is energy. People with very keen intelligence always have a lot of mental energy, while those with dull intelligence have less. More energy to the brain gives greater awareness, while less energy gives diminished awareness. With exposure to this greater energy from the galactic center, mankind has begun to expand its awareness and appreciate the subtler workings of nature.

This is the way both Sri Yukteswar and the ancient scriptures explained planetary evolution. They said that when we're in the closest position to this galactic center, we're in the stage of relative enlightenment, which is called *Satya* or *Krita Yuga*, or "The Age of Truth." It's the time when many more people are aware of the spiritual nature of this world.

When we are farthest from the center, we're in *Kali Yuga*, or "The Dark Age." In Kali Yuga we have no awareness of the spiritual basis of reality. At that time, we see our bodies and all matter as the ultimate reality. Heaven is hardly conceived of except in human terms, like a court with a king on a golden throne and many courtiers. All spiritual truth is reduced to dogmas, forms, institutions, and laws. This is all a part of Kali Yuga thinking, where people are hypnotized by the thought of the solidity of everything.

Hegel, the great German philosopher, said, "All that is real is rational. All that is rational is real." To him reality had to be something you could analyze and reduce to a formula. This is typical of *Kali Yuga* thinking.

Now we've come into a new age, *Dwapara Yuga*, or "The Age of Energy." It actually began in 1700 AD, but there's a bridge of 200 years coming into and leaving the age. During that transitional period you had whole new ways of thinking—Democracy, Social Revolution, and the Industrial Revolution. Finally, at the end of the Nineteenth Century we entered Dwapara proper, and the kinds of changes in human thinking since then have been extraordinary.

My parents were born in the 1890s, and at that time there weren't any cars or airplanes. I've often quoted the story that at the turn of the century the head of the United States Patent Office suggested to Congress that they close down his office, because everything that could possibly be invented had already been thought of. Then suddenly science opened up an entirely new view of the universe, and new vistas are emerging all the time.

Because of Einstein's discovery of the Law of Relativity in about 1900, science is much closer to a spiritual view of reality now than it was a hundred years ago. We thought science would make atheists of everyone, but instead scientists themselves are beginning to think that there is a consciousness behind matter. They obviously don't think of God in merely dogmatic terms, such as a Being with only one son who lived in Israel two thousand years ago. The thought, however, that there is a consciousness underlying everything is coming very much to the forefront of scientific thinking. This is because they see that the essence of matter is energy, and that there seems to be an innate awareness in that energy. There's a rationality in it, but it goes so far beyond reason. You can't think only in rational terms, analyzing and defining, and hope to arrive at ultimate truths. You can't make mental definitions and expect them not to change.

This is a part of the charm of the book *Alice in Wonderland,* which, though a children's story, was written by a famous mathematician, Lewis Carroll. He had an intuitive awareness as a student of mathematics that definitions don't stay fixed. Thus when he wrote about the croquet game, for balls he used hedgehogs that would run away, and for mallets flamingos that would suddenly turn up and look at you. He was trying to tell us through this fantasy that the universe doesn't stay fixed.

There's an intriguing discovery I've read about recently in which scientists have found that when they split an atom, the electrons don't seem to be separated at all. There's no perceptible connection between them, but as one electron moves, another one moves in the same pattern. There's some sort of yet undefined web that exists on a level of energy. Physicists are beginning to think that it looks very much as if energy is, in fact, a manifestation of consciousness.

They can't yet prove this, however, so they're very conservative in what they accept. This causes a big split in our thinking, because we don't want to be biased and support something we feel but can't prove. Science tries to rigidly exclude emotion, which is essentially the correct approach. Finding truth isn't like a horse race, where you root for a horse to win because you've bet on it. Science says you have to see things as they are, not as you want them to be. They make the mistake, however, of concluding that feeling has to be biased emotion, and therefore rooted in likes and dislikes.

The truth is that no great discovery can be made without intuition, which in essence is calm feeling. Only with intuition can you perceive reality as it truly is, can you know you are a part of everything, or feel your connection with all life. This is something that scientists are increasingly coming to understand. Einstein intuitively perceived the Law of Relativity in an instant, but it took him the next ten years to explain it mathematically so others would accept it. Even then, only ten scientists in the whole world knew what he was talking about. The power of intuition is beginning to be appreciated in the sciences. When we can bring together not emotion and reason, but feeling and reason, then these two produce profound insights and divine consciousness.

As planetary consciousness continues to evolve—in other words as the yugas ascend—we will move past Dwapara Yuga, which gives us an awareness of energy. All the discoveries of this age are essentially manipulations of energy. Today we're just at the beginning. The discoveries that lie ahead of us are enormous, but all of it will be based in one way or another on an awareness of energy as the underlying reality.

As Dwapara continues, however, and the age progresses, people will begin to become more aware of the power of consciousness. They'll begin to understand that consciousness precedes energy, and that with our own minds we can direct energy to accomplish things. This will be the hallmark of the next age, *Treta Yuga,* or "The Age of Mental Power." We know this principle to some extent even now. For instance, Yogananda's Energization Exercises teach us that by will power we can send energy to the body. "The greater the will, the greater the flow of energy," as Yogananda used to say. It's consciousness acting on the energy, and energy acting upon the muscles that tense them. As we go deeper into that thought, we realize we can ultimately send energy to manipulate even the events around us.

This principle is also demonstrated in what gamblers talk about as "beginners' luck." The simple explanation for beginners' luck is that people who are new at something such as gambling don't yet recognize the obstacles involved. There's not a division in their consciousness where one part of their mind says, "This is what I want," while the other part says, "Oh yeah, what are the chances?" This inner conflict produces a kind of mental static that blocks the flow of energy.

If you could put all your will into making something happen, and not have any conflicting doubt, you would find that your will is enormous. Will power isn't just generating the energy—it's also removing the obstacles that prevent that energy from being effective. Otherwise it's like pushing on two sides of a door. You can exhaust yourself, and the door doesn't move. That's why they say,

"Faith can move mountains," and this is why masters are able to perform miracles. They know that when they will something, they must send out all their energy, and there's no conflicting energy blocking it.

I saw an ad in a magazine once for somebody who was supposed to be channeling an entity. I had to laugh when I looked at his picture because the man's face was all screwed up with the effort. When Yogananda did miraculous things it was effortless, because there were no conflicting thoughts. He just sent out a thought, and even though he had tremendous will, there was never any sense of struggle. It's not as if God had to get all worked up to project the universe—it just happens very naturally.

There's a book that Yogananda loved called *The Life Everlasting,* by Marie Corelli. It's an inspiring story, a spiritual allegory, about a woman's search for divine love. At one point in the book, the heroine has gone through all sorts of tests to work through the things within her blocking her progress. When she has eliminated these blocks, she's told by her inner guides to look up at a rose on a tree and ask it to stoop down. She does this, and the rose immediately stoops down. Life itself adjusts to the desires of one whose consciousness is clear.

In Treta Yuga, the Age of Mental Power—an even higher age that comes after Dwapara Yuga—people live much more on the level of conscious awareness, and are able to direct things through the use of mental energy. When archeology shows us the artifacts from ancient civilization, what we often see is that they didn't have anything but the simplest places to live, such as caves. What we're really seeing, often but not always, is that there were civilizations that didn't need houses. Nature itself was clement, because the predominant consciousness at the time was peaceful. That's why, as described in

Autobiography of a Yogi, when Sri Yukteswar asked Babaji to his ashram, he replied, "We are people who like the shelter of trees." They didn't live in houses, and still today there are saints who don't need houses.

A woman in India told me about her guru, who lived very simply in the forest. Once when a number of his disciples were with him, there was a heavy downpour of rain, but it was completely dry around them. It was as if he had created an astral umbrella, though he didn't say anything about it. When you have that inner power it's a very small thing to ward off the rain. You can put out the kind of energy to prevent rain or to cause rain, or even to change the seasons.

So in Treta Yuga people are aware enough to be able to manipulate energy with will power. Still, they don't yet necessarily have the degree of mental control that enables them to act in attunement with God's will. There still is warfare well into Treta Yuga, because people's emotions aren't yet under total control. They haven't yet fully learned to attune their consciousness to the divine will. By Satya Yuga, the highest age, we will have learned that.

In *Satya Yuga* there will be a much greater degree of Self-realization. This doesn't mean there won't be people whose consciousness is negative or dark. We're talking of a relative state of realization and purity of consciousness, because we're still living on a material plane. Even in Satya Yuga, we're still quite far from the center of our galaxy. There are whole galaxies that are far more evolved spiritually than our own, just as there are others that are far less evolved. Even in the depths of Kali Yuga there are still a few masters around, and in the heights of Satya Yuga there are still a few evil people. It's rather that in Satya Yuga relatively more people have an enlightened awareness and use it, so that warfare is no longer a problem at that time.

An encouraging thing about the cycle of the yugas is that the Dark Age, Kali Yuga, is the shortest, while the highest age, Satya Yuga, is the longest. Satya Yuga has a cycle of 4800 years ascending, and 4800 years descending as we move closer and then farther away from the center of the galaxy. Treta Yuga has a span of 3600 years, Dwapara of 2400, and Kali of only 1200 descending and another 1200 ascending as we once again begin the long journey towards the center of the galaxy. As you see, the whole cycle takes 24,000 years, and this cycle repeats over and over again.

We have now entered the upward swing of Dwapara Yuga. It's interesting to think what was happening at the point where Dwapara was descending into Kali Yuga. What would be the natural tendency of a civilization that was coming down from higher levels of spiritual awareness and losing its ability to use mental power? It would be to turn toward magic, wouldn't it? You would still be left with the memory of past civilizations being able to influence everything with the power of the mind, but you wouldn't understand how to do it. Eventually you would try to recapture this lost power by doing everything with incantations and magic.

In fact, if we look back to what was happening historically during descending Dwapara, we see that the ancients were people not thinking in terms of moving earth with bulldozers, but of doing everything with incantations. I felt very strongly when I was in Egypt that the entire civilization at the time of descending Dwapara Yuga had fallen into black magic. There was a darkness over the land. But further back in time, I felt something much more uplifted. When I was in the

Aswan Dam area, I had a very strong feeling that I'd lived there long before in a higher age—I could imagine lush greenery everywhere, and that it had been a very simple, harmonious time. It had a very different vibration than what I'd just seen of the bas-reliefs on the temples that were created in descending Dwapara.

The time we're coming into now makes it especially interesting to see the struggle between Kali and Dwapara ways of thinking. The Kali Yuga approach is to think in terms of form: of institutions, dogmas, fixed ways, "either/or" Aristotelian ways of thinking. Dwapara opens the door for a new approach to reality: personal, fluid, and one that accepts the possibility of different perspectives coexisting. Because we are just at the beginning of Dwapara, however, old ways of thinking are still very prevalent.

For example, scientists say that beings couldn't possibly visit Earth from outer space because the nearest star, which shows no signs of having planets, is four light years away. They say it isn't possible to travel at the speed of light, and therefore it would take them much more than four years to get here. "Why," they ask, "would anybody launch himself into space for that many years with the uncertainty of finding anything?" To the old guard it doesn't make sense. They also say that any planet with life on it is probably much farther than four light years away.

The Sun, which we think of as far away, is ninety-three million miles from the earth. It takes eight minutes for the Sun's light to reach this planet, while it takes four years for the light of the nearest star to get here. Four years—that's a long time. So according to science, it's not possible for people to go from one solar system to another because of the incredible distance and time involved.

But Yogananda said the opposite. He said that there are other ways of space travel besides just using physical instruments and space ships. There is also a great deal of evidence of Earth actually being visited from outer space. Lots of credible people have said they've seen UFOs, so it's starting to wear thin when science declares, "It absolutely can't be, so therefore it isn't." There's been a big attempt to put down the whole idea, but the abundance of evidence is starting to convince people otherwise. Too many people of reputable position and experience in observing objects in the sky, like pilots and air controllers, are coming forward and talking about it. Many people are also talking about having been abducted.

There's a movie about what happened in Roswell, New Mexico, where a flying saucer crashed in 1949 and was seen by many local residents and military personnel. They saw the beings on the ship—some had been killed in the crash, and some survived briefly. They even took movies, but these were suppressed by the government. Today enough people who saw the crash and examined the bodies are coming forward so that the evidence is starting to come out. The beings looked similar to us only smaller, but they didn't have the same cardiovascular system that we have. It was more like that of plants.

There's no reason why other physiological and biological systems couldn't work. We have a carbon-based system here, but it doesn't have to be. Master said there are planets on which people are as tall as from here to the moon—that would mean a huge planet and probably not physical bodies like ours. I believe Master also said that even on the Sun there are entities whose bodies are made of gas.

The thought that we can't travel to other planets, or even other galaxies, is not necessarily so at all. I've not made a great study of visitors from outer space, because I think it's absurd to assume that because a being is from another planet, he therefore knows more than our spiritual masters. Anybody who knows God, knows God. You don't have to be from another planet to know more of God. These beings who visit Earth don't necessarily have great spiritual wisdom—they're engineers, pilots, and technicians. It makes me smile when I read some of the messages from those supposedly from outer space telling us to love one another. Haven't all the masters said we should love one another? They're not masters— you don't need them to teach you.

But as we move into Dwapara Yuga, we're coming into an age when religion, art, and science are going to be much more on a level of energy than of form. Energy is fluid—you can manifest a loaf of bread, then dissolve it back into a stone because there's no actual difference between the two. It's only that they've taken on different forms for the moment. This new awareness is going to change our thinking in many different fields. We're going to have much more understanding of the need for intuition as opposed to exclusively using the rational process.

It will be reflected in the practice of medicine and the healing arts. I think that in a hundred years from now, people will look back on so-called modern medicine as a kind of superstition. When I was in Mexico in 1945 someone told me a very interesting story. His father had a hacienda in the country and employed many farm laborers from nearby villages. One day one of the workers was riding on the tongue of a wagon, slipped off, and fell underneath the wheels. One of the wagon wheels went over his head and cracked his skull open, leaving his brain exposed. Though the man was still breathing, when the doctor saw him, he said, "There's nothing we can do for him. He can't live." His friends asked, "Can we take him to his village?" The doctor replied, "Yes, take him. There's no hope. You might as well take him home and bury him." The man was taken back to his village, which was quite a distance away. Six months later he walked back to the hacienda without even a scar.

That kind of knowledge—to heal someone of such an injury—is something that our modern medicine doesn't have. A lot of the discoveries made by science, such as quinine, are based on knowledge of simple tribes. Where did they get that knowledge? Some of it may have been handed down from ancient times, but much of it is based on intuition. So in Dwapara Yuga we're going to find that, across the board, people are thinking more in terms of using their intuition rather than relying solely on reason.

This explanation of the yugas gives meaning to the seemingly random events of history, the endless rise and fall of civilizations. It is also increasingly substantiated by science. What are the lessons we can personally draw from understanding the yuga concept? Yogananda said these cycles are the "eternal rounds of maya." As mankind, one by one, escapes from duality, he awakens to realize his unity with God. To the spiritual devotee, in a sense, it doesn't matter what yuga we find ourselves in. We need to tune in to the higher octave of the time in which we live, and use it for our spiritual development. Dwapara Yuga is the Age of Energy, and Yogananda came at this time to give us techniques of energy to help us achieve Self-realization. Let's use these techniques well, and transform our inner world into a higher age of divine truth.

Chapter Two

Worshipping God as Divine Mother

"Be suspicious of too much use of the intellect, because ultimately it's your intuition that gives you the real answers."

In our culture today we don't have much awareness of the Mother aspect of God. I didn't know it existed until I read *Autobiography of a Yogi* back in 1948. I was so moved by the book that I took the next bus from New York to Los Angeles to meet Yogananda. He was lecturing at the Hollywood Church at the time, but when I went there, they said his appointments were booked solid for the next two months.

I felt pretty bleak about this, and was standing there sadly wondering what to do next. I suppose I needed to learn humility, because until then the doors had opened easily for me in everything I'd tried to do. It was good karma, perhaps, but here was the one thing I really wanted, and the doors seemed to be closed. I thought, "Maybe I'm not ready," which was a novel thought for me at that time!

Then I decided, "I'll just meditate, pray, and wait until I can see him." Just as I was about to walk out of the church, the secretary who was arranging the appointments came running up to me and said, "Since you've come such a long distance, I'll ask the Master if he can fit you into his schedule."

Yogananda agreed to see me. When I went into his interview room, he said to me, "I want you to know that I didn't see you because you've come from such a long distance. There was a lady here last week who came from Sweden, and I didn't feel to see her. I will see people only if Divine Mother tells me to, and Divine Mother told me to see you." This was my first personal experience with the concept of God as Divine Mother.

As I think back, I wonder whether a saint would have said, "I will ask the Heavenly Father if I should see you." Somehow the Mother aspect of God is more personal. You have confidence in the mother, whereas the father has more to do with law, justice—he's a bit more removed. Yogananda used to say, "When you pray to God as the Mother, pray, 'Naughty or good, I am still your child. You must receive me.'"

Someone introduced our topic today as "God in the Form of Mother," but I would like to correct that thought. The Mother aspect of God can indeed be visualized as having a form, because we need form before we can reach the formless state. But really, God has no gender; God is not literally a mother. When people manifest any aspect of human nature, it isn't necessarily that those people are like that. You see a girl smiling sweetly, and you think, "How sweet she is!" Two minutes later she could be in a rage. What we manifest is not our own self. It's an aspect of a consciousness that's there, and, just like a cloud in the sky, it passes. People can be sweet or harsh, but in every case, they manifest something that is not their own.

Yogananda made a very interesting statement in *Autobiography of a Yogi* that most people gloss over. He said, "Thoughts are universally, not individually, rooted." That is to say, whatever level of consciousness you're on, that kind of consciousness will manifest through your thoughts. You are the product of your actions, attitudes, and the things that you've developed during this life and many previous lifetimes. You are the product of all of that, and yet you are none of those things. You aren't jealous and vindictive, or kind and forgiving. Those are qualities that are coming through you, perhaps, because you've opened yourself up to those aspects of a much greater consciousness.

It's good to keep this in mind for the basic reason that, if we want to realize who we are, we have to go beyond the ego. The ego is our friend and our foe, depending on how we use it. It's our friend if we say, "I want to grow spiritually. I want to get out of this ignorance and out of my human capacity for suffering. I want to find a state of divine consciousness."

One of the great mistakes that we find in this country today is victim consciousness. This leads to the kind of thinking that says, "I am the product of my environment, a product of the way I was treated as a child, of the way my boss treats me." The problem here is that it puts the blame on other people. We need to realize that we have a choice: We can develop the attitudes that will keep us immune to the storms of life, or the attitudes that allow us to fall subject to those storms. It's like saying, "Here I am in a house, but there's a storm outside. I don't like storms because they make me unhappy, and I'll open the windows to prove it." The other attitude is to close the windows and make sure you're comfortable within.

It seems quite obvious that we have control only over the way we react to circumstances. Essentially all spiritual teachings say this: You need to develop those attitudes that render you immune to adverse conditions, no matter how life treats you. There are some people who have had tremendous adversity in life, and yet somehow they come out as heroes and heroines.

For example, sometimes other people can hurt you very deeply. What will your reaction be? If you hate in return, does this make you happy? Is hatred a solution? You may get even, but I don't think you'll feel happy even if you do. You suffer when you hate, but you're happy when you love. Therefore, strictly in your own self-interest, you should love. It's the only thing that makes sense, because otherwise you lose twice—you're hurt by others, then you hurt yourself by hating. Why not give the lie to their negative attitude and say, "I love you anyway."

When you are in a giving mode, you grow. But when you are receiving egoically, with great concern over how people are treating you, you contract and suffer. To put it on the bluntest level possible—you aren't that important to other people that they should think that much about you anyway. Why not just say, "I am who I am, and I choose to be happy." Nobody can make you happy except yourself. How others treat you may feel good, but that's not making you happy. If you can say, "I am complete in myself. It doesn't matter how people treat me," then you can begin to find unshakeable happiness.

One great help in doing this is to think of God as somebody to share all your thoughts with. Because we're human, we spend a lot of time thinking about other people—what they said, how they treated us. Why not have the thought that you're relating to someone who can't possibly let you down? Why not relate first and foremost to God? God is your own Self, and knows and loves you better than any person possibly could.

People make a mistake in their concept of God. When I meet self-proclaimed atheists, I don't accept that this is really what they believe. What they're rejecting are definitions of God that have been dumped on them. They say, "I can't believe that God is a policeman up there judging me, or that He is just a human being when I see this creation with hundreds of billions of galaxies. It just doesn't make sense."

But it does make sense to think of an impersonal consciousness, or, taking it down to a more personal level, of the source of those things that make you happy. You do feel better when you love, when you try to include other people's happiness in your own. These things are fundamental to human nature. They can't be different for one person, or even for beings on other planets, because all of creation is part of the same consciousness.

Yogananda gave us a beautiful definition of spiritual vision: "Center everywhere, circumference nowhere." Our understanding has evolved from the time when everybody thought the Earth was the center of the universe, to now when people think the universe doesn't have a center at all. The next point of spiritual evolution will inevitably be the realization that every atom is the center of the universe. From any perspective you take, you can understand everything. If you want to look at the universe as an artist, you can explain everything in artistic terms. If you want to think of it as a scientist would, you can explain it from that center.

You are the center of the universe—each one of you. We need to learn how to relate to that center within us, and in other people. We need to realize that each person is a center of equal importance, so that we don't become self-centered and shrink down. You can take a period on any page, shrink it for the next thousand years, and still you won't be able to reach the point where it has become nothing. It can't become non-existent. It can become infinitesimal and shrink down to the size of the smallest electron, but it cannot cease to exist. You cannot cease to exist. You are a part of that eternal, omnipresent consciousness.

What happens when you limit your sensitivity and compassion? You become smaller in your own consciousness by being selfish, and you suffer. Just as people hate to go to prison, they also don't like being in an ego because it's confining. When the ego thinks only of its own happiness, it becomes its own enemy. But when you think expansively and realize that this little center that is your ego is the same center that is in all, in every atom, then you raise your consciousness from the human level to the divine.

In thinking of ourselves as this little dot of ego, we are taking a *gyanic,* or discriminative, approach. If you want to go according to the philosophy of Vedanta, you think, "I am God. I am that Infinite consciousness." There's also truth and inspiration in this approach, but somehow it tends to be cold. I've noticed from years of living in India that many swamis who go by this philosophy become egotistical. They have too much of the consciousness that says, "I am everywhere." The ego in that way is an obstacle. If you use the ego to say, "*I* want to find liberation. *I* want to get out of this suffering," that's good.

This is what we have over the lower animals, who in some ways are more spiritual than we, at least in their intuitive flow. Mankind has reached the point where we begin to say, "I don't like to suffer," whereas animals don't yet know that they're suffering. We have sufficient awareness to say, "I want to know how to get out of it," though it may take us a long time to reach that point. Most people think, "If I can only get this or change that one thing, then I'll be happy."

Much of modern self-help is on that level. It's as though you're in a little room of the mind, and you're suffering because of some complex you're trying to overcome. You read a book that tells you how to get out of that room, how to overcome that complex, and you feel good. You're no longer bothered by that problem, but after a while you look around and find that you're just in another room. You go on from room to room, but that's not growth—it's just change. You need to get out of that building altogether. That can only be done by divine awakening and awareness on a soul level, not by the intellect or self-help systems.

The truth is that without God's help it's not possible for the ego to get rid of itself. One good way to draw God's help is to talk to Him in an "I and Thou" relationship. It's not that God is separate from you—God *is* you. The only difference is, you aren't God. Do you see the distinction? The ocean can say, "I'm the wave," but the wave can't say, "I'm the whole ocean." The ocean sees that it's all those waves, whereas the wave is still small. It can't say, "I, as a wave, am the whole ocean." It has to take gradual steps and say, "I am that salt water of which the whole ocean is composed." It's hard to affirm, "I am God," and then go into the bathroom in the morning, look into the mirror, and say "This is God." It doesn't quite work somehow, though it's true.

God is your own higher Self, but it helps us to visualize Him with a form. In a very real sense God is neither father nor mother, but in another and broader sense He is *both* father and mother—and beloved, and friend, and anything you want Him to be. Even if all of us here define God as mother, it still will be a different image to each person. It can't be otherwise. There may be a particular image of that infinite consciousness that everybody worships, but even so, it will mean something different to each person according to his or her training and life experiences.

Just as a home might mean something comfortable to a person who has been brought up in a typical way, it might mean something altogether different to somebody from an orphanage. The words we use are only symbols. But behind those symbols, we can have a personal relationship with God in which we confide more, trust more, and feel unconditionally loved and accepted.

Whatever way that we try to define God will be limited. Once I met somebody who was trying to persuade me to join his church. I replied to him that there are many ways of approaching God, but this man wouldn't buy it. So finally I said, "There's one thing we both have to accept. However each of us defines God, we're both wrong." He couldn't refute that, so he had to let it go. We *are* wrong. How can we be right? How can this little mind conceive of something so vast, that has created hundreds of billions of galaxies and all the little microbes and bacteria? Everything is a part of that consciousness.

There was a disciple of Yogananda who kept asking him to give him *samadhi,* cosmic consciousness. He kept after him until finally one day Yogananda looked at him very intently and said, "Could you take it, if I gave it to you?" The disciple stood there for a moment, then looked down and said, "No."

Omnipresence is no joke. It takes a lot of deep meditation and great loyalty to find the path that is right for you. You won't get it by frittering your time away and flitting from one flower to another. After reading *Autobiography of a Yogi* and meeting Yogananda fifty years ago, I haven't for one moment had the question, "Is this my path?" It is. That question was settled fifty years ago, and I don't have to ask it again. We need that kind of loyalty to what is the right thing for us.

But in our relationship with God, it's a lot easier to love God in human terms, and especially to love God as that which is nearest and dearest—the Mother. To most human beings this mother aspect is the most precious because you feel with the Divine Mother that, no matter what you do, She still loves you. She won't judge you. No matter who you are, She's your friend. She's on your side and will always forgive you.

Certainly all of us err at one time or another. You don't want to feel guilty in the sense of guilt-ridden, but you do have to accept the fact if you've made a mistake. Otherwise you're going to go out and do the same thing all over again. What makes things spiritually wrong? It's not that society defines it as such, but because your own nature tells you it's wrong.

Here's a simple example: If at a party I see that there's not enough cake for everybody, am I going to rush in there and get mine? Most people might think that way, and they may feel good in the short run. But there's something inside that says, "It would have been nicer to share it, or let somebody else have it." As we grow more sensitive over many incarnations, we reach the point where we find happiness comes not from getting the cake for ourselves, but from seeing that somebody else got it. As we grow spiritually we want to include the happiness of other people in our own, even to the extent of not wanting it for ourselves, but wanting it for them. You find there's real freedom in realizing that nothing outside yourself makes you happy, but that your happiness is something that you can carry with you into sleep, into work—all the time.

All of this ties in with that expression of God that we call the Mother aspect. In human nature basically two things rule us—reason and feeling. In most of the world today there's been altogether too much use of the reason and not much use of feeling. We think that in order to be scientific, we must exclude feeling, because it prejudices our mind. But, in truth, feeling is the only thing that gives you real understanding. People make the mistake of confusing feeling with emotion. Emotion does confuse the understanding; likes and dislikes confuse the understanding. They're like waves on the sea. When you've got waves, you can't see the moon reflected clearly in the water. But when the water is calm, then we see the undistorted reflection.

Now if it weren't for our feeling aspect, we couldn't achieve true understanding. Reason by itself is an inadequate tool—it can show you a hundred directions to follow, and they all make good sense. What is it that finally tells you which direction to take? Feeling. Be suspicious of too much use of the intellect, because ultimately it's your intuition that gives you the real answers.

Those scientists who go only by reason are the lesser scientists who do minor experiments, or sweep up the pieces from the great discoveries that others have made. But *great* scientists go more by feeling and intuition, or as Einstein put it, "the sense of mystical awe." For instance, Einstein perceived the Theory of Relativity in a flash, and then had to spend ten years working it out so that he could explain it to others. Many great scientists have had this experience.

I read an interesting book recently by George Abell called *Talks with Great Composers*. Abell lived in a time when he was able to have interviews with major composers and ask them about the creative process. Brahms, for example, said that only minor composers create out of their own minds, but that great composers receive. They hold their minds up in a state of openness to allow inspiration to come to them. We need to understand that in any area inspiration comes through receptivity and intuition. When you intuitively feel what is right, you *know;* you don't have to think anymore. Of a thousand choices you simply know the right one.

But remember, intuition is not just another level of ignorance; intuition is soul knowledge. A lot of people think they have intuition, but it's just emotions. Intuition is calm feeling. Thousands of years ago Patanjali gave the classic definition of yoga: *"yogas chitta vritti nirodha,"* that is, "Yoga is the neutralization of the vortices of feeling." *Chitta* is the feeling aspect of consciousness. When that feeling is disturbed, as it is in most human beings, they don't perceive things clearly, because their likes and dislikes influence them.

Women tend to go more by feeling, and men more by reason. In the last analysis, we aren't women or men, but are influenced by the cosmic feminine or masculine principles working through our bodies. Whether man or woman, intuitive people have a strong feminine quality in them because they go more by the feeling of the heart. They consult that feeling, and then they know what to do. Usually, however, women are more intuitive than men, especially when tuning in to other people.

Many times, for example, a man will ask his wife what she thinks about a new business partner. She may say, "I don't know, but I don't feel good about him." The man says, "Oh, you and your intuition." But frequently it turns out after a few years that she was right, and the person proves untrustworthy. It's not safe to say you're infallible with intuition, but do listen to it. If you have an intuitive feeling about something, go more by that, and increasingly you will be guided in the right direction.

When it comes to looking at the heights to which we can aspire, I think that the Mother aspect of God is not only beautiful and inspiring, but I would go so far as to say that it is essential at this time in our evolution. Our whole society has become too bound hand and foot with reason. It needs more feeling and love. The thought that you understand a thing by not feeling, that you're being scientific and facing the truth if you're cold, is wrong. You don't face truth that way because truth itself is love.

It's only when you can develop the heart quality that you are able to perceive things as they really are. It's only when you empathize with others and don't judge them from afar that you can truly understand them. You don't want to stand outside the window of life looking in and not be touched by what's going on. You want to go into the building and find out what's really happening there. You want to be involved, not with agitated emotions, but sensitively. Empathize with the people you meet, know them from inside, and try to feel what their aspirations are. Each one of us is unique and extraordinarily complex.

I was recently reading a book by the great English novelist, Jane Austen. I was fascinated by her analysis of human motivation because it showed that each person's actions were driven by hidden desires, and underneath those there were still other motives. You go down this ladder, and finally you find there's really no bottom to the basement. But the interesting thing was that in her heroes and heroines there wasn't hidden motivation. The difference was that they were clear.

I finally got to the point where I was tired of looking at people on the basis of ego-motivation, because basically we're united by one thing. The ego unites us on a certain level, but we're all really united by the fact that we aspire to goodness, and to the spiritual potential we have inside.

There's a strange but beautiful story about John Dillinger, who was called Public Enemy #1. He died in a police shoot-out, and by his body they found a note saying, "I've been much misunderstood. In this body beats a very loving heart." Even Dillinger, who was full of hate and violence, believed in his own basic goodness, because it exists in everybody. The worst Mafia gangster has God inside—he just needs to work harder to uncover it. We all have that aspiration to become who we know we really are. For a time we may think we'll get power by killing people, or get happiness by becoming rich, but bit by bit over incarnations we weed away those false goals, because we find they don't give us what we really want.

When you can get out of the ego and out of the thoughts "I must have this, or do that, or achieve this recognition," then you realize, "I'm complete in myself." When you can reach that point—and it doesn't come except by meditation—then you suddenly find, "Now I know who I really am." It's like peeling an onion. The onion isn't completely peeled until there's nothing left. Think of yourselves as an onion, if you like, because you have to peel away all those false self-definitions.

Now divine grace is very important to this process, because if you're trying to scramble out of a well, you need somebody to help pull you out. You need somebody who is out of that confined consciousness to bring you to a sense of freedom. Otherwise you just struggle backwards and forwards, and you never get out. By loving God, you allow grace to enter into your life.

Your job is to find fulfillment in your Self in the midst of all the storms going on around you. You can do that by keeping a strong awareness of the presence of a divine friend, of Divine Mother, whose attitudes are perfect. People may not understand you, but God, especially in the aspect of Divine Mother, understands you. People may betray you, but God will never betray you. Your own higher Self couldn't betray you because She *is* you. There is no way She could betray you, unless you let your ego come in and betray yourself from that level.

We need to think of God in such a way as to give us a sense of confidence that She's on our side. We need to think of God as Mother, and to think of that Mother aspect as an ideal of feminine qualities—not the emotions, but that calm, always forgiving and accepting energy. It's easier to define this as feminine, rather than as masculine, energy. Finally, we need to realize ourselves as both feminine and masculine.

Great saints are androgynous. Yogananda was on a train once and, as you know, he had long hair. Because his consciousness was so balanced, sometimes he looked like a mother, sometimes a father. A porter was walking up and down the aisle looking at him, and finally said, "Is yo a man, or is yo a woman?" Yogananda answered in a very deep voice, "What do you think?"

The woman saint of India, Anandamoyi Ma, was very feminine in a sense, but also very masculine. I spent a lot of time with her in India, and in the way she walked and stood, she looked like a general—very determined.

When she spoke it was with great confidence. She was a balance of both, and yet she was neither.

We are like that too. We aren't limited by our physical forms, our personalities, or even our problems. We shouldn't take our problems all that seriously, because they aren't who we really are. Work with them as you would with a dull saw that needs sharpening, or a dirty microscope that needs cleaning. Don't get all upset about it, but don't refuse to accept that it's dirty.

There's a story about a Catholic, a Baptist, and a Christian Scientist who all died and went to "the wrong place." They were trying to figure out how they got there. The Catholic said, "I must have missed Mass one Sunday." The Baptist said, "Perhaps I wasn't fully immersed when they baptized me." Then they asked the Christian Scientist, "Why are you here?" He replied, "Oh, but I'm not."

You have to accept where you are, but then—and this is where confidence, love, and faith in the Divine Mother aspect of God come in—think of the love, not the judgment. That's what uplifts you. If you can say, "I've made these mistakes, but naughty or good, I'm your child," then you get the strength and the sense of perspective that gives you the power to say, "All right, I'll try again." Never say you've failed. No matter how many times you do fail, don't accept failure as your definition. The world will try to define you by your faults. You define yourself by your aspirations.

Yogananda used to say, "If ever you say, 'I've failed,' then you've lost it, at least for that lifetime. But if you can hang on, and even at the moment of death, say, 'I *will* succeed,' then you can overcome."

There's a beautiful story from the life of St. Francis. There were three men in the area of Assisi who were criminals. They were stealing and doing all sorts of bad things, to the point where the townspeople were so angry that they went after them with pitchforks. These men sought sanctuary at one of St. Francis's monasteries. Now, St. Francis was away at the time. The monk in charge was so scandalized that these evil men should seek protection in a house of God when they'd lived such ungodly lives that he drove them out with virtual imprecations. The men left with great anger, cursing him as they went.

When St. Francis returned later on that day, the monk told him in outrage of the audacity of these evil-doers, daring to come to a monastery for help. St. Francis was properly outraged in his turn, not with the criminals, but with this monk who had sent them away! He commanded him on his vow of obedience to go and look for them and bring them back.

When they came back, St. Francis greeted them, saying, "Brothers, why do you live the way you do? You're not happy. It's not only other people who are suffering from your bad deeds, but you are suffering." He began talking to them of their own potential for goodness to the point where they became converted and ended up becoming monks. According to the chronicle of the time, they lived very holy lives and died in a state of grace.

This was possible because St. Francis helped them to see their own divinity. Who are you to doubt your divinity? You're insulting yourself. That's the worst kind of insult you can deliver. You must have faith in your own goodness because it's potentially there, no matter what you've done. You should get rid of a guilt complex, not by sweeping it under the carpet, but by saying, "I am yours, Mother."

When you love the Mother in that way, it's so much easier than thinking you're going before a judge. You know the judge is likely to punish you, but the Mother will help you. She may give you some hard lessons, but that's Her business. You know She does it with love. No matter what tests you go through in life, know that it's for your good, and don't complain.

Finally, we come to what this is all about. The more you can bring yourself to that attitude where you completely trust Divine Mother, the more you will be open to God in your life. When you have that understanding, you can open yourself to the infinite compassion and forgiveness of God as Divine Mother, and you can develop those qualities in yourself. That's why it's necessary to forgive other people, because in that forgiveness you, too, become softer. It's as though you've got this little seed that can't grow because it's had concrete poured on it. You have to break up that concrete so the seed can grow. You've got that seed of divinity within you, but all this concrete of ego, desires, self-importance, and strain to reach for things blocks its growth. In this world we're trained to think we must fight and compete for what we get.

Yet it's a world based in consciousness. Consciousness produced the energy that produced this world, which is seemingly made of solid matter. Yes, you can approach the solid matter with a sledge hammer, or you can get back into that flow of consciousness, and somehow matter itself adjusts to who you are.

The kind of attitudes and, above all, the kind of feelings that you radiate are sooner or later what you will become. This is a law. So think of God not as distant, but as very close. Talk to God. It's easy to talk to the Mother, because She understands you. She doesn't justify your mistakes. She doesn't say, "Yes, I think you're fine," when you're really not fine at all. No, She's wise, but She's also the friend of that seed of divinity that's trying to come out—not of the concrete that's keeping that seed locked in the solid wall. She wants what's best for you.

Here's something that I've experienced—because you can't be on the spiritual path without learning a few things over the years. I've seen again and again that when things in life happen that seem to be the worst possible things, if you can say, "This is coming from you, Mother, and I accept it," then suddenly it all becomes just the right thing, the only possible thing. On the other hand, the things that you thought *should* happen for the best outcome, in hindsight prove to be the worst. The more you give your life to God in this spirit, the more you will find that whatever She gives you, it will be right for you—for your growth, for your ultimate happiness.

There's a story of a king who had a chief minister he was particularly fond of because of his wisdom, loyalty, and good counsel. This minister's motto in life was, "Everything that happens is for the best." Due to the king's particular regard for this minister, all the other court advisors were very jealous and were always trying to undermine the king's faith in him. He didn't listen, but the poisoned words entered the king's subconscious and had a little lingering power.

One day the king was out hunting in the forest, and that day the chief minister, who was usually with him, wasn't present. The king had an accident with his bow and cut off his thumb. When word of the accident got back to the chief minister, he calmly said, "Everything that happens is for the best." The other ministers with great vindictive glee reported to the king, "Look what he really thinks of you! He said it's for the best that you lost your thumb." The king allowed himself to get angry and threw the minister in prison, where he remained for many months.

The next time the king went hunting, he rode off by himself in pursuit of game and was captured by some cannibals. They were about to sacrifice him to their gods when they saw that he didn't have a thumb. They couldn't offer their gods an imperfect sacrifice, so they had to let the king go.

When he returned to the palace, he immediately had his chief minister released from prison, and said to him, "You were right after all. If I hadn't lost my thumb, I would have lost my life. But what about you? You had to suffer in prison for all those months." The minister replied, "Yes, Your Majesty, but if I hadn't been in prison, I would have been with you. And as you know, I haven't lost my thumb."

So don't doubt. Don't you think the God who created this vast universe, who created you, knows what He's doing? Don't worry too much about how the world is going. Divine Mother knows what She's doing. Maybe we have hard lessons to learn, but they're for our good.

You will have more of that consciousness if you think of God not only in the *form* of Mother, but as that Infinite Mother in every atom, in every cloud, in your own heart, everywhere. Think of that motherly aspect of the Infinite Consciousness that created and loves every single being in this universe because every being is a part of the Infinite One. If you love the Mother in that way, if you love God in that way, then you will find a remarkably sweet relationship developing in which you have a real awareness, not just an imagination, that Mother is always with you. She watches over you, takes care of you, and hears the yearnings of your heart. If you hurt your thumb and say, "Mother, it's bleeding," you'll feel Her response.

I had a wonderful experience this way many years ago when I was at Mt. Washington. My parents were living in France, where my father was working as the chief geologist for Esso in Europe. As a boy I'd gone to school in Switzerland, and had come to love Swiss chocolate. Since my parents were living nearby to Switzerland, I had the thought that it would be nice if they would send me some chocolate. But it was such a trivial desire that I kept forgetting to ask them about it whenever I wrote. Then one week before my birthday, I remembered it again, and thought, "Oh, Divine Mother, it's too bad I didn't think of it. I could have asked them to send me some for my birthday. Now it's too late, but never mind." I gave the desire to Her.

A day before my birthday I got a package, not from my parents, but from someone in the Hollywood church, where I was a minister. She didn't know it was my birthday, nor that I liked Swiss chocolate. With the package was a note saying, "I saw this chocolate in a store window. I don't know why, but I thought to send it to you." It was a box of Swiss chocolate.

If God can take care of us in such trivial ways, won't She take care of us in important things, in life-and-death situations? Divine Mother will be more instantly responsive if your consciousness is attuned in this way. What I'd like to do in America is try to get people to think of God more as the Divine Mother. We need God. We have gotten away from devotion. It will be easier for America as a whole, which has a natural kindness in its soul, if we love God in this personal way. Even though God is impersonal, it's through the personal that we can reach that vastness and find oneness with the Infinite. God bless you.

Are there any questions?

Q: *I feel that there is a real violation going on across the whole planet against the Mother, with violent entertainment and movies, and violence against women and children. It seems the male energy is having a hard time receiving the Mother, the female energy, to balance itself. What can we do?*

A: Here's the way I look at this sort of thing: Problem consciousness doesn't produce solutions. Solutions come only from the superconsciousness. If I think of what's wrong, I don't get the answers. If I think that there must be an answer, then it comes. There's always going to be resistance to any new wave of energy. Nobody has ever done anything really important on this planet who hasn't had to fight a lot of resistance in this great ocean of maya.

I was touched by a response that Buckminster Fuller once gave. I happened to hear him on the radio, and the interviewer asked, "You talk all over the world, but nobody ever listens. Doesn't this discourage you?" It was rather a cheeky question to ask someone of eighty-four who had been doing his best to spread new ideas, but I loved his answer. He said, "Not at all. Any new idea requires at least one or two generations to become recognized."

This is true with the consciousness you're asking about. It's not so much the violation we need to think about—that's to be expected. Anti-feminism is also partly a natural response to excessive feminism. Whenever one side becomes polarized, the other will resist. So I say the cure for it is not to get angry, not to fret too much about it, but to put out more positive energy. God knows what He's doing with this universe. It'll change in its own time. We have to love more, that's all.

Q: *Would you agree that loving yourself is one of the first steps to being able to love others?*

A: I've heard this, and of course I agree, but I also disagree. Obviously in some sense it's yourself you love when you love others. You don't learn to love humanity by loving a neighbor who keeps dumping his garbage over the fence, or who keeps singing at the top of his voice. You have to love in a general way, and this comes by meditating and feeling that love in yourself. Then you can give it to everybody without needing a reason to love. If you love people because of what they are, will you dislike those people who aren't that? Will you feel hatred for people who are selfish? You have to get deeper in your understanding of what you're loving. Ultimately it's a projection of the love you have in your own heart that comes through attunement with God. You don't get it by affirmation or by changing your mind about things. It comes from a superconscious level.

The problem with this concept of loving yourself first is that I don't want to love this ego. I want to love that which this ego can become. I don't want to love what I am, but rather my potential. I have the potential to be kind even if I act unkind. To say, "I'm going to love my unkindness because it's me," is to deepen one's delusion. So I would love that highest potential that you see in yourself, but not you as a human being with human faults. Love yourself because you are a child of God, and because Divine Mother dwells in your heart.

Q: *How do you know what's appropriate to say to somebody who's asking you for advice?*

A: If you think of it too much in the way of rules when you're faced with the need to give advice, then you've got this mental file to go through, and it doesn't work. What you need to do is have a basic consciousness that is attuned with an intuitive flow within yourself. From that intuitive flow, sometimes even to your own surprise, you find that you're saying, not what you intended, perhaps, but what's appropriate and helpful.

Naturally we all come into situations where we think, "What shall I say? How shall I answer?" I've found that in such situations, it's best to be in my heart. Don't prepare an answer in advance, but prepare yourself. You do this by developing intuitive openness, and then the inspirations come. When somebody asks you something, if you're centered in the heart, you'll know how to respond. If you make mistakes, join the club. We all make mistakes, but this is the direction in which to go. Eventually you'll make fewer and fewer mistakes, until finally you get it right.

There was a woman in Italy who asked me for counseling. I didn't want to give her any advice, because I knew she would reject whatever I said. But she insisted, and finally I thought, "Okay, I'll tell her." So I said a few things as generously as I could, but they were a little difficult to face, and she became frozen. I said, "I hope you're not angry." She replied rather aloofly, "No, I'm just disappointed." I had to leave it at that. Two years later she finally said to me, "What you told me was what I needed to hear. Thank you."

So often even if the immediate reaction isn't right, it will sink in. If your advice is true, it will register in their subconscious mind, and eventually they'll understand. So don't worry about how people respond at the moment. Very often it won't be the response you would have liked, but if you've said the truth with charity and without condemnation, they'll take it inside and dwell on it. The very fact that you didn't hammer on it will mean that they will be more likely to look at it. If they are to change they will, but it's between them and God.

You are the only responsibility that the universe has placed on your shoulders. You're not responsible for others. What you can do for other people is your free gift to them. Never allow yourself to think that because you've given someone advice, he owes it to you to be grateful. You do it for yourself, your larger Self, and you should do it in freedom. I think possibly the thing of greatest spiritual value is that which will give you true freedom inside. If when you give advice you don't force your thoughts, but just offer them, then you will feel freedom and God's smile in your heart.

Q: *In my prayers and meditations I ask God to help me drop the ego, but it doesn't go. What's your experience with this?*

A: Dropping the ego is not easy, because it's all that we know until we are in divine consciousness. Don't get upset about your ego, because it's such a sneaky thing. When I first came to my guru I had a lot of intellectual pride and was praying just as you do. After a time, I began to feel that I was making progress and was feeling very good. One day I woke up to find that I was becoming proud of my humility! The ego is such a subtle trickster.

I think the best thing to do is to say, "So what? What else is new?" Think more of God, and give Him everything you do. Give Him the fruits of your actions. That's what the *Bhagavad Gita* says to do. You have to act and take responsibility for what you do, but give the fruits of your labor to Him.

The next thing is to think of Him or Her as the Doer. (I say "He" when I *talk* of God because that's convention.

I say "She" when I *think* of God because that's my feeling. So I pray to God as Mother, but I talk of God as Father.) Feel that His power is working through you. This feeling won't come quickly—it takes incarnations for most people.

Once I said to Yogananda, "Have I been your disciple for thousands of years?" I asked him this because another disciple had had a vision of being with him thousands of years ago. His answer was, "It's been a long time. That's all I'll say." I asked, "Well, Sir, does it always take so long?" He replied, "Oh, yes, desires for this thing or that take people away from the path time and again. They learn their lessons and come back."

So, even after you come on the spiritual path, it's a long process. Most people have no conception of how long it takes to reach the point of even being on the spiritual path, or even wanting truth. It takes, as Yogananda put it, "very, *very,* VERY good karma even to *want* to know God." But once you're on the path, you're virtually liberated. Granted it can take a few incarnations, but if you have the desire for God, that desire has to be fulfilled. All desires have to be fulfilled. Once you're consciously aware of the desire for God, the most deep-seated desire of all, it will guide you bit by bit over many detours to final realization.

But why waste all that time? When you come to the point of ecstasy and have the experience of God, then suddenly you realize all the lives you ignored the Divine. You think, "How much time I've wasted!" Then the tears come, but they aren't tears of regret. They're tears of joy, for at last you know what you're here for. At last you know that finding God is the only thing that life is all about. All those other thoughts were just a waste of time.

Your job is to know God, and your heart will never know peace until it knows Him who is your true Self.

I had an inspiring experience watching the movie, "The Sound of Music." There was a moment in that movie when the Baron, the hero, and Maria, the heroine, suddenly realized they were in love with each other. At that moment there was absolute stillness. Then they expressed their love for each other and kissed, but the real moment of love came in silence. True love can only be experienced in absolute motionlessness, breathlessness, and ecstasy. There is no love outside of God, because there is no ecstasy outside of God. There is no breathlessness or stillness outside of God. Seek that kind of love which doesn't send you dancing through the streets singing in the rain. Seek that kind of love that makes you absolutely still.

That point will come in your meditation when you become enrapt, and you know what you were made for. You know who you are, and nothing can shake you from it ever again. Live for that moment, because it will be yours. It has to be yours, because you are a part of that. Live in that thought, and you will know freedom sooner rather than later. There's only one thing you were made for, and that's divine love.

Chapter Three

A Tribute to Yogananda

"The legacy of Paramhansa Yogananda is that consciousness which will change you and make you as he was."

To offer a tribute to Paramhansa Yogananda is to offer a tribute to all of you, because a great master comes into this world not to show us how great *he* is, but to show us *our own* potential. If you look back over the history of the human race, you'll see that all the great changes that have occurred haven't come from a rational level, or from the intellect, but from a higher intelligence—the superconsciousness. All the great discoveries, the great inventions, and above all the advances in consciousness have come quietly, almost without notice at first. They virtually never come from a governmental level, but from people—from grassroots movements and small groups.

The great changes of history brought by Buddha, Jesus Christ, and other great saints and masters have come into this world without any fanfare. Buddha was born the child of a king, but he renounced his kingdom in order to become a wandering mendicant. Jesus was born in obscurity in a lowly manger. All great saints have come humbly, because the ways of God are humble. When we read *Autobiography of a Yogi*, we hear about the classes that Lahiri Mahasaya gave on the *Bhagavad Gita*, and we assume that there were large crowds there. Yet when you go to Benares and see the balcony on which he taught, you realize it was only big enough for perhaps fifteen people. The great movement of Kriya Yoga started with only a few people.

In the *Bhagavad Gita* it says, "Out of a thousand, one seeks me. And out of thousands who seek me, one here and there finds me." The search for God is not a mass movement. It's not some sort of mania that seizes a nation as in the time of the Nazis, when suddenly everybody was thinking in an aggressive way, or in the time of the Renaissance, when everybody was painting and sculpting. It's not some fad or some new mass awakening, though our minds would like this because we tend to think in terms of outward things.

I remember somebody wrote to Yogananda at the death of Mahatma Gandhi and suggested that he return to India in its hour of need. They wanted him to lead India on the path of spiritual righteousness. In my heart I thought, "Oh, wouldn't that be wonderful! What a great destiny that would be." I responded this way at the time because I was thinking as a person who had been planning to become a playwright. I was thinking of drama—how perfect it would be for the human race to see the greatness of spiritual truth.

But the wonderful thing about God's way of doing things is that it's quiet. God doesn't impose some external reason on your will or discrimination for following a religion or for doing anything. Even now I've often wondered why Yogananda's work isn't going out to millions. It could, and someday it will just as Christianity did. In some ways we should be glad if it happens, but the plain fact is that the day Christianity became the state religion was the day of its beginning descent. It was no longer as great as it had been, because it had become official, institutional, and powerful. God always works quietly.

Jesus said, "Go into your closet, and meditate and pray." The spiritual masters tell you to do these things quietly on your own. Yogananda talked about churches that would be small, where a few serious, sincere devotees would gather together to commune with God and to experience Him in a deeply personal way.

I remember when Master was lecturing at Hollywood Church, it held 110 or 115 people and was always full when he spoke. Then an Evangelist minister came to Los Angeles and gave a lecture one block from Hollywood Church. Thousands flocked to hear the evangelist. I thought, "This is what Master's work deserves," and yet perhaps that's not what mankind is ready for. It's always going to be a small group of people who have the power to really change our civilization. As they say, "One moon gives more light than all the stars." One enlightened soul, or even one sincere seeker of God and truth, will have more influence over humanity, over his country or town, than thousands of other people making a lot of noise, but all just for ego satisfaction. Those kinds of religious teachings that tell you how to become successful will always attract large numbers.

What Master and all the great saints come to bring to us is the inner realization that divine enlightenment—union with God—is what it's really all about. In fact, you can divide the human race into two basic camps: One is swollen with great numbers of people; the other has just a small scattering. The one seeks its fulfillment and gratification outwardly. The other seeks within.

A great master really comes for two purposes. The first is the qualitative: He comes for his disciples, to enlighten a small number of people who really want the truth. But he also comes for a second purpose and a very important one—the upliftment of the entire human race.

A great master can do this, whereas ordinary teachers cannot. Spiritual teachings differ from one age to another, because the human race as a whole needs different aspects of truth at those particular times.

When Yogananda came, he didn't just tell people to withdraw, meditate, and pray. He also came to show us how to use divine teachings in this world, so as to advance in an outward as well as in an inward way. In his interpretation of the *Rubaiyat of Omar Khayyam*, he emphasized that if we want to do good, we should align ourselves with divine love and divine law. Even with all the goodwill in the world, we cannot impose wholesome reforms on humanity if it isn't ready, nor if divine law doesn't endorse that kind of change.

You have to do what is right. A master could come in with miraculous power and change everything, but it wouldn't help people. People wouldn't be ready for it. It's like tearing down a broken-down tenement and putting up a beautiful apartment building in its place. If the same people move in, it often quickly becomes another broken-down tenement, because the people weren't ready to take care of it. We have to change people's consciousness. People get out there waving flags and shouting angrily for peace, but without peace in their consciousness how can this come about? Unless and until you can change people's hearts, the scene will not change—it will go on as ever.

Thus Yogananda's life had this twofold purpose— qualitative and quantitative. He was always upholding and promoting both of these goals. Living with him, it was quite surprising to see how very practical he was. He once told me that it was his idea to put the gearshift on the steering shaft of a car. He drove into Detroit with a prototype, and they picked it up and took it over from there. He also said it was his idea to put lids on toilet seats. These are things that you wouldn't expect a master to think about, but he was interested in practical improvements. At the same time, he wanted to work with human nature and ability.

Yet when he was with the disciples, his talk was very different from what you read in his books, or from what you would imagine. It was even very different from the way he spoke outwardly. The most important thing that he said to us again and again was to be in tune with that power that he brought. Most people weren't ready to understand this, but it was through that power that our lives and consciousness could change. We couldn't do it by ourselves.

I remember a very interesting story of one of the women in his ashram in Encinitas. I knew her, and she was a radiant, joyful person. But she met some other spiritual teacher who claimed to have certain powers. Yogananda didn't use powers. He had them, and he did use them in his early years, but later he stopped because he saw that it wasn't the way people would really be helped. Their hearts had to be changed—it wasn't enough just to blow their minds, so to speak.

This woman was impressed by the new teacher, who told her that if he was meditating on a mountain, he would suddenly come out of his meditation to find himself on another mountain top. Who knows whether it was true, but what would it matter if it was? At any rate, this woman decided that she would follow him, and told Master of her decision. With respect for her free will he said, "Very well. I will withdraw my ray." She came back a year later for a visit, and all the light that had been in her was gone. It's amazing how we can change according to what thoughts, feelings, and states of consciousness are coming through us.

I remember another woman who was radiant, full of love and joy, with a very beautiful personality. She began going through a difficult period, and I was to meet her at the train station. I waited and waited, but I didn't see her get off the train. I went into the waiting room to look for her, but there was only one person there, and I didn't recognize her. Then I thought, "Oh, it must be she." Her features had all changed because her consciousness had changed.

We have to change our consciousness, and we can't do that by our own power. You see, we are locked in an ego. How are we going to get out of its grip? The ego is already infected with the very disease it's trying to get rid of. You need a doctor, but you need somebody who will do more than just tell you what to do and give you medicine. You need somebody who has found the way out of ego. The way a guru works is that often he doesn't speak at all, or very little. Perhaps he'll just say one word, but it's his consciousness that changes you.

There's a story of a saint I met in India, Narayan Swami, who worked in that way. A woman came to him and asked, "Please will you pray for my son? He's taken our family inheritance since my husband died, and he's squandering it on women, gambling, and drinking. I'm afraid we'll end up poor and that he'll be ruined." He said, "All right. I'll talk to him." When the son came, he began chatting with him. He asked him what kind of drinks he liked, and the boy told him. "Oh," the saint said, "this whiskey is much better." He asked him questions about his gambling, and he told the boy, "Oh, this place is much nicer."

The boy was delighted, and went home and told his mother, "Your swami agrees with me, not with you. You call him your teacher, but then you'd better listen to me." The woman was crushed. The next morning, however, the boy got up, went out and got a job, settled down, and never went back to his dissolute ways. What this saint did was work on his consciousness. He was giving him terrible teachings, advising him about the best whiskey, but when he talked like that the boy relaxed. He was no longer hostile, and he accepted the saint's influence. In that process of acceptance, he took into his consciousness something of what the saint was really trying to do for him, which was to get behind the scenes—to change his attitudes. As a result, the boy was completely transformed.

This is an example of how the saints work. It isn't so much their books or their actions—it's their consciousness. This is what Yogananda used to do in the ashram in talking with us. He emphasized again and again, "Be in tune." The more in tune you are, the more you will find yourself going in the right way. You'll understand what you should do. You don't need a lot of guidance—this is a path of *Self*-realization. It was always surprising whenever anybody went to Master for instruction. Knowing the way counselors work with people today, you would think that he'd talk at great length, ask them about their childhood, analyze it all carefully, and then say, "Ah, do you see this? Do you understand why you behaved that way?"

He did none of that. Sometimes it was discouraging trying to get his advice until you began to understand what was going on. He would give you just a word or a sentence. But I've found that those sentences had such power that I've meditated on them for the rest of my life trying to understand more and more deeply what he meant.

I've written in *The Path* about a man who came to Master with all these intellectual questions. After a while Master said, "Love God." The man thought, "He's sort of missed the point, hasn't he? I've got all these very deep questions, and that's all he's answering?" So he went on and asked a lot more questions, and Master said a bit more strongly, "Love God!" He thought, "Everybody's got his problems, but I'll try once more." So he started in again on another list of questions. At a certain point Master got up and said, "LOVE GOD!" and walked out of the room. This man had such a shallow understanding that for years he used this story to show that even saints have their problems and don't understand certain things.

What Yogananda was saying, if this man had had the humility to understand, was that only through love for God will you have understanding. Without it, you won't be able to comprehend anything deeply. Divine truth is not something you put together like a jigsaw puzzle—it's a revelation. It's something that is given to you. Sometimes he did give long dissertations, and sometimes he gave long answers when he felt that the situation demanded it. But the most important thing was that he always wanted us, and encouraged us, to understand from within.

I have hundreds of stories about Master, and I've told many of them in *The Path*. In fact I hope to write another book someday in which I'll tell many more. Yet when people ask me to tell a story about him, it's strange but I can't think of one, because for me the stories are always tied to some truth. When a point needs to be made, then I can remember all kinds of stories to illustrate that truth, but I can't remember it just as a story. I think this is because I never thought of him as a personality. We should all try to think of him as much more than his personality, because that died many years ago.

I'm one of the few people still living who knew that personality, and it was a dynamic, beautiful, fantastic personality. I've never met anyone in my life so powerful, so joyful, so full of love, so magnetic. He was a powerhouse, and yet he was so sweet and lovable. To think of him as a person is to be overjoyed just from that simple association with the memories of one who lived for a while on this earth. Yet, he was so much more, and that is what is still with us today, and what is right here in this room now. That is what is spreading this work bit by bit. It's not spreading by mighty waterfalls, but by one soul at a time, maybe a hundred souls at a time. Each one individually has to recognize his or her need for this truth and absorb that within.

No institution is going to give it to you, nor any official dogma or other people representing an organization. I myself can come here and talk about these things, but it will help you only to the extent that you recognize it within yourself. Truth cannot be taught—it can only be recognized. My endeavor all these years has been to try to put these truths in a way that will help people to recognize them, but finally it comes down to a heart recognition. Finally it's just that and nothing more—when you know truth in your heart, you change.

There's a lovely story that one of Master's disciples, Louise Royston, told me shortly after his *mahasamadhi*, his physical passing. He was buried at Forest Lawn, and all the nuns were praying around his body. Many of them were weeping. Louise Royston, who was an older woman, was standing a little outside the circle of disciples and feeling his presence inwardly. Suddenly she distinctly heard Master's voice say with great scorn, "I'm not in *there!*" He wasn't in that tomb or in that body.

We have to recognize that he lives in our hearts. God lives in our hearts, and He uses channels to help make these divine realities more dynamic to our consciousness. Otherwise, if we think of God only in the abstract, it's very difficult to comprehend. It's when we see divine love, compassion, kindness, and even good humor manifested in human form that it becomes real for us.

Jesus is somebody whom most people love, but they find it difficult to think of him as an ordinary human being who could sneeze, tell a joke, tease somebody, or do any of the things that ordinary people do. With the common view of Jesus as somebody who was always standing around grieving and weeping for people's sin, frankly, I don't think that many people would be drawn to him. Are you going to be attracted to somebody who's always feeling sorry for you because you're so terrible? No.

He was a man of joy. He was magnetic. Just by glimpsing him, people followed him and thought, "This is what I want." Do you want more sorrow? Do you want more self-condemnation? Do you want to feel how bad you are? No. What he gave people was a sense of hope for themselves. He wasn't an angry young man, though that's what the Bible often makes him seem to be. He was a man of great joy, wisdom, and of power to change people's lives.

This is what we read in the stories of great saints everywhere. Think of St. Francis, who is considered by many to be the most perfect of all Christian saints. He was a saint of joy. The Catholics today depict him as a saint of sorrow, but he had the joy to transcend the suffering he was given, and to realize that nothing is important except the divine joy of the soul. This is why Yogananda called him his patron saint.

There is a lovely story of St. Francis called "The Secret of True Joy" that could also be the story of Yogananda. There is so much similarity between the two, although Yogananda had more power, and St. Francis was more gentle. In the story, St. Francis and his close companion, Brother Leo, were walking in the winter through a snowstorm, trying to reach a monastery before it got too late. St. Francis called ahead to Brother Leo, "Do you know the nature of true joy?" Leo replied, "No, Brother Francis, instruct me." Francis said, "If we come to this monastery, and the monks receive us with open arms, that isn't true joy. If they bring us in from the cold and snow, and warm us by the fireplace, that isn't true joy. And if they give us good food to eat and nice beds to sleep in, that is not joy."

"But if when we come there and knock on the door, they open it and say, 'Get out, you reprobates,' and they throw us into a snowdrift, and refuse us entry, or love, or comfort, or food, note well, Brother Leo, that is true joy." It's not that suffering is true joy. This is where the Catholics go wrong. What St. Francis was saying is that we must have that kind of joy that isn't touched by anything outward. If we truly have joy, we are able to accept whatever comes, whether it be a fireplace, warm clothing, and a nice bed, or a snowdrift. True joy doesn't depend on any outward circumstance.

You see, the emphasis has been lost. Now the emphasis is on the sorrow, as if that were joy. How can you call that joy? People mistakenly think the story means that if you suffer enough in this world, you'll get to heaven and be able to be smugly self-righteous, while all the others who enjoyed a warm fireplace go to the other place and get too much warmth. This is not the spiritual teaching, and this is why great masters have to come into this world again and again to correct misconceptions of the spiritual path.

People think that those people who channel entities or write esoteric things must be therefore be highly enlightened beings, but there aren't that many great masters that come onto a planet. Usually what happens is that, after a few centuries everybody agrees that someone like St. Francis was a great saint, and they all say, "This is what *he* taught." Perhaps he taught that then, but what the masters teach now in *this* time is the right teaching for us. It's not that it's different, but it gives a different emphasis.

Someone asked me a question recently about the Essenes. I said, "What do we really know about them? They had a certain teaching, but mostly it's been interpreted for us by scholars." Don't read too many books. Don't get too involved in all the different theories of what different people in the past have said. We need to tune in to the way God is talking to us now. When Master was a young man, he made a comparison to Swami Sri Yukteswar between his work and some other spiritual work. I presume it was the work of Ramakrishna, because that was contemporaneous with them, and Ramakrishna was a great master. But Sri Yukteswar said, "Why do you make comparisons? This is the way God is playing through you and me."

God plays different songs through different great teachers. But when you find a particular teaching that deeply satisfies you, then you don't need to read about everything else. Stick with your own way, even if other teachings may be equally true. Great teachers certainly don't contradict each other, though in an outward way there may seem to be contradictions. This is because one teacher will be addressing the needs of one group, and another the needs of another.

There's another important thing, and that is that great saints come into this world with different degrees of divine power. Even a saint who is fully liberated, a *siddha,* hasn't the same power as an *avatar*—one who is born in this world after achieving that liberation. That is why when Lahiri Mahasaya saw Yogananda as a little baby, he said, "As a spiritual engine, he will carry many souls to God's kingdom." Yogananda had that kind of power that comes with being an avatar. Very few avatars are born in this world, so don't discount the power that is in this path—the power to change souls.

I would say that the real proof of it is in the faces of the people who live Yogananda's teachings. I've seen people come to Ananda with their faces filled with lines of worry and care. Within weeks they're transformed because of that power. It's not because of a good lecture that they heard, but it's something that happens by osmosis.

A mistake I used to make many years ago was that I thought my job as a disciple was to bring people to my guru, and then I could wash my hands of them because he would take over. But it doesn't happen that way. I remember being in India at a time when Master's work wasn't doing well. The people there didn't appreciate who he was, and they were reading other books, and drawing from other teachers. When we were leaving, one of the nuns said, "What will happen to this work?" Another one said affirmatively, "Master's here. Master will take care of it." I said, "Master's been here for forty years, and what has he done? He can't do it except through you and me. God needs human instruments."

It's not the divine way to send down a ray, and then suddenly everybody sees the light. No, it radiates outward from individuals. Somebody came to Ananda Village once and said, "What wonderful people you have here!" I said, "If you met one or two of them you might say, 'What wonderful people.' But when you're speaking of a whole community, you can't say that. We don't have exams that people have to pass with flying colors to get the degree 'Wonderful Person.' It's what they're doing that makes them wonderful."

I didn't add, but easily could have said, "You should have seen them when they came." You should have seen me when I came. We change when we get in tune with something higher. Look at the clouds at sunset. They're beautiful—radiant, golden, orange, pink, sometimes with even a touch of green. But then the sun sets, and only minutes later those same clouds can be gray, dark, and ugly. Then you understand that what made the clouds beautiful was that the sun was illuminating them.

You will be beautiful to the extent that you are in tune with that divine consciousness. That beauty doesn't come through reading a lot of books. It's brought forth by being in tune, and through your techniques trying to feel that attunement, trying to feel that God and Guru are doing everything through you. The more you act and live that way, the more you find yourself becoming free. It's not as though you become a slave to somebody else's will. The will of God is to free you according to your own nature. Each one in this universe has a unique song to sing. The masters are here only to help you to know who you are, and they give you the power to realize your true self.

It's like a stained glass window. At midnight it doesn't look like stained glass because it's all black. Before dawn you see a little bit of light, and it looks gray because the colors aren't distinguishable from each other. But, when the sun comes up and shines through it, all those colors become beautiful. The more you become in tune with that divine power, the more it shines through you, the more you become who you really are, in blazing color and glory.

Most people think they're just being themselves, and often say, "I just want to be me." There was a song I heard recently, "I love myself just the way I am." I think that's a mistake. If we go deeply enough this is valid, because the way you are is divine. But if you're speaking of the way you are as your personality, or as the person you see when you look in a mirror, then I have to say that, frankly, I doubt it. There may be a few people in this room who in fact are radiating from within outwardly to that extent, but mostly we take our beliefs, our personalities, our reactions, and all those things that we define as our personalities from other people.

It's like watching somebody come out of a John Wayne cowboy movie, and you see him walking like a cowboy with bowed legs. It takes a while to shake off that hypnosis. This is how we are. Why do Americans act like Americans? Why don't they act like Indians? Why don't they act like Slavs or Egyptians? It's because they've been brought up in this country. You take on the influence of your environment to that extent, but we need to get deeper than that. We have to know that who we really are is that divine spark.

Yogananda came for the quantitative upliftment of many. But the real work that Yogananda came to do, that any great master comes to do, is the qualitative work that is done on the individual soul. If out of a crowd they can find one, then that's what they're really here for.

I remember one time, Oliver Rogers, an older disciple, came to Mt. Washington, and said to Master, "You know, I heard you in Boston Symphony Hall in 1920, but I lost track of you, and only recently heard of you again. It's strange that, throughout your talk, I thought you were looking right at me." Yogananda said quietly, "I remember." Imagine that! Out of five thousand people, he remembered that he'd seen one soul that he knew was ready. He had looked at that soul, looked into his eyes. Though the soul didn't change quickly, still he couldn't get that power out of his system, and finally he came back. Oliver was a house painter, and I remember Master saying to him, "In the astral world you will be painting flowers." He used to say, "God chooses those who choose Him." If you choose God deeply, then He will take care of you.

I remember my first meeting with Master. I had read *Autobiography of a Yogi* in New York—it was a marvelous experience for me because I hadn't known anything about these things. Before reading it, I didn't know where to turn. I was ready to give up everything, go into seclusion, and try to find God through meditation in South America where the living was cheap. I was confused, but I was deeply searching. I didn't want to go to church, because it wasn't giving me anything. I read in a book that you should meditate, but I didn't know how. I remember sitting cross-legged and cross-eyed on my bed not knowing what to do. Then I saw *Autobiography of a Yogi,* and it was really a miracle for me. I took virtually the next bus across the country, non-stop, and went to Los Angeles where he had been lecturing in the church there.

When I met him, he said, "Divine Mother brought you here. Divine Mother told me to speak to you." I was so amazed that Divine Mother would take that interest in me, but She does. When you lift one arm up, She drops two to pick you up. When you take a little step, She opens the path and welcomes you. She doesn't always make it easy, because She wants to test your sincerity, but you must understand that She knows your thoughts, She knows the heart of everyone individually. God is infinitesimal as well as infinite. God is not only in you, He *is* you. Behind the scenes, behind your thoughts, behind your feelings, God is there. If you listen, and if you ask for help and guidance, it will be given to you.

I remember the time Master asked me to come out to the desert retreat at Twenty-Nine Palms to work with him on editing the books he was writing. The first one was the interpretations of *The Rubaiyat of Omar Khayyam.* We've recently published the edited version that I did because years ago he had asked me to work on it. He said, "I prayed to Divine Mother to tell me whom I should take to work with me, and your face appeared, Walter. I asked her twice more, and each time your face appeared. That's why you're going."

I know that Divine Mother, having created all the galaxies, all the incredible laws of science, and produced this whole fantastic show, is definitely not stupid. She knew I wasn't ready to edit that book then—I was twenty-three years old and inexperienced, even though my plan had been to be a writer. She was planting the thought in my mind, so that later I could do it. Master said to me after that long job, "I predict that you will be a good editor some day." He knew it wasn't the time yet, but the thought that Divine Mother should take a personal interest in me, and tell him to bring me along, shows the infinitesimal nature of Her love.

There was a disciple named James Coller who Master described as "like hot molasses—too hot to swallow, but too sticky to spit out." He was somebody who was always breaking the rules in one way or another. He was the minister of the Phoenix Church, and once was driving back to Mt. Washington to see Master. He got very hungry along the way and stopped at a restaurant to eat. When he found that all they had was hamburgers, he thought, "Well, Master won't know," and he ate one.

When he got to Mt. Washington, Master met with him and was giving him advice for his work in Phoenix. Then he paused at the end of the session and said, "Oh, by the way, when you're on the highway, and you're hungry, and you enter a restaurant, and all they have is hamburgers, better not eat." He knew. But later he said of this man, "He will find liberation in this life. I don't know how, but Divine Mother says so, so it has to be true."

Divine Mother is very conscious of you, and especially of your soul's needs. She will help you, but She will help you more if you ask from Her that which She really wants to give. Master put it in a beautiful way when he sang a certain song in Bengali. Somehow he gave me the power to remember his words. I even remembered this song well enough so that ten years later when I went to India and learned Bengali, I realized that I had learned it exactly right. The song was, "Oh devotee, I can give you salvation, but don't ask my love and devotion. If you ask for those, and if I give them away, I become poor because then I give myself away. So ask of me any gift, ask of me even salvation, but don't ask me for my love." Of course, the meaning is that Her love is what you really should ask for.

Ask for love, ask for God's love, ask for Divine Mother's love. There's nothing else worth praying for, even salvation. It's not important whether you're living in this world or in another world. Be in love with God. There's a beautiful thing that St. Theresa of Lisieux said: "I want to go to hell because I want there to be at least one person in hell who loves God." Have that longing for devotion. If you pray for anything, pray for devotion. If Master brought anything to us, above everything else, it was that love of God.

He didn't love people just as people—he loved God in people. True, he was a good friend to everybody. He was loyal, charming, and amazingly considerate of others. He was so good as a human being. He was totally human, but human in a perfect way rather than what we think of when we say, "I'm only human," which means "I'm imperfect." You might say of such people, "They are not yet human," because they haven't yet fulfilled their potential as human beings.

But the main thing he saw in everybody was his or her divine potential. He used to ask me to serve guests who came to Mt. Washington, and then he would have me demonstrate the yoga postures. Incidentally, I became expert at the yoga postures in one evening. I wasn't very good at them, but he had a group of us demonstrate them to some visitors. In his presence, suddenly I found I could do them perfectly. From then on, I did them quite easily. I even wrote a book on the subject and taught yoga postures along with meditation. All of this came about by a moment in his company.

I remember another disciple, Norman, telling me how he learned to do the lotus pose. He had never done the pose before, but Master just pointed his finger at him and said, "Do the lotus pose." He was afraid he couldn't, but he thought, "I'll have faith and do it." He found he could do it easily with no problem. Master had that kind of power, but he didn't usually demonstrate it. He didn't say, "Lo! From now on, you shall be a good yogi." Rather, in his presence things just happened naturally.

But the most amazing of all was the way people changed in his company. That power to change others is still present today. This is what I really want to bring to you—the realization that you, too, as a disciple, must be an instrument for that power, and not just expect a few others to do it. Whatever inspiration, or blessings, or joy you feel in your heart, offer that to others. Let it radiate outward from who you are because, as it does so, you yourself will grow. The light blesses those through whom it flows, and it will not flow by imposition. It will flow as you invite it to do so. That's how this work will spread to many people. Each one becomes a catalyst so that everybody you meet in some way is affected by it.

I've seen this happen again and again. Often people sitting next to me on a plane say, "Gee, I just feel good sitting next to you." They don't know why, but I know why. It isn't me—it's Master's presence. When you're with people, don't just descend to their level. I don't mean you should stand up on a pulpit and pontificate, but quietly in your own mind send them blessings. Ask that this person be helped, or that that person be uplifted. You can do it because Master can do it through you. He came to bring that power. It's like those seeds that Johnny Appleseed planted all over the country, so that in time apple trees grew up everywhere. That's what Master's mission is—to change our lives, and through that change to transform many other people's lives as well.

In your meditation, in your devotion, don't put yourself down. Don't say, "Why don't you come to me?" or

"Please help me not to be such a horrible person." Realize that you have that potential to be another Christ. If it doesn't happen in this incarnation, it will happen. If it doesn't happen in ten incarnations, it will happen because it's your divine destiny. It's what you were born for.

The wonderful thing about a great master is that he comes to show us who we really are. In his presence, suddenly you begin to think, "I'm not all that bad after all." Don't preen yourself. If you do, you've still got a few more lessons to learn, which is okay. It takes time for everybody, but the truth is there should be great humility in the realization that this power isn't yours. It's something that can be given through you, something that you can tune in to and become, but as long as you're thinking it's your ego, then you're limited. It won't work. Be humble. Be little before God, but don't belittle yourself. Always feel that inside there's that germ of divinity which is your reality. That germ is waiting to sprout and become a tree, and eventually it will become a great oak tree spreading its shade over many people. It's like a banyan tree growing into a whole forest. Whatever simile you use, remember that it's the divine power that will enable you to do that.

The greatest thing that Yogananda came to bring was that power which is silent but very active in people's lives. He won't be able to touch others unless it's through those who are in tune with him. This power would die if there were no disciples. If he had just been somebody who lived and wrote a few books, in a generation his mission would no longer have any life. We have to carry forward that spark ourselves, and in that way it will reach out and touch others.

The legacy of Paramhansa Yogananda is that consciousness which will change you and make you as he was. There is no greater glory that you can give him than to become more and more like him, not in his mannerisms, but in his devotion, his joy, his ability to see everything as Divine Mother's play. Nothing else matters.

Once we were helping him into his car because he was having trouble with his knees. He said to us, "You're so kind doing all these things for me." We said, "Oh, Master, when one thinks of what you're doing for us, what is this kindness?" Then he smiled so sweetly and said, "God is helping God. That's His drama." Depersonalize it. Realize that it's all the divine show working through him, working through you, working through everyone. If you want to change this world, that thought alone will change it. Be in tune with him, and realize yourself as an instrument for his love. Joy to you!

Chapter Four

Kriya Yoga—The Universal Science

"Yogananda brought Kriya Yoga not only as a means of finding success, but of finding divine enlightenment. This indeed is what life is about."

Truth can be likened to a pyramid—from its pinnacle the highest expression of truth radiates, while its broad base gives strength and stability. In a society like that of India, which for thousands of years has had a broad-based acceptance of spirituality, even atheists know a great deal more about spiritual truth than most Westerners. I've been amazed by the number of people in India who tell me they don't believe in God, and then go on to demonstrate that they do. They can't get away from it—it's a part of their whole upbringing. They don't necessarily define God in terms of somebody like Krishna who is blue and plays the flute. But the thought of an infinite consciousness is so ingrained in them that it's impossible for them to reject it.

Because the highest expression of spiritual teachings throughout the ages has usually been found only at the pinnacle of the pyramid, the result has been that very few people reached it. Spiritual teachings were often esoteric, and those few people who received them would seek solitude in the mountains or monasteries. This has happened often in the history of religion. Even though the truth is there, new spiritual movements don't spread far or last long, because they don't have wide acceptance.

Without a broad base the pyramid sways, and people can't find their way to the top because the path is too difficult.

When Paramhansa Yogananda brought the teaching of Kriya Yoga to the West, he understood the need to create a broad-based pyramid that was accessible to many. In fact, Kriya Yoga is the central core of that pyramid because it helps to magnetize the inner spiritual spine, and thus bring everything into alignment with a higher reality. This effort to bring life into attunement with higher realities is what India has done for thousands of years.

The Vedas, the ancient Indian scriptures, had such a broad base that they even give you spiritual techniques, mantras, and ceremonies to help you fulfill all your worldly desires. If you want fame, or power, or success, or a good husband, wife, or children, the Vedas show you how to accomplish it. They are a surprising concoction of teachings to help man to become, and to develop, that which he wants.

In our purist idea of scriptures, we might ask, "What kind of scripture is this that fulfills your worldly ambitions?" The rationale is that if you use a ceremony with spiritual power to become wealthy, you'll remember that your wealth came from the scriptures. If you gain it through some technique learned on Wall Street or Madison Avenue, you'll be grateful to Madison Avenue. If people begin to see that they get what they want from the scriptures, they'll gradually turn their minds to God.

I remember a disciple of Yogananda who was worried about his own worldly desires. He asked Master, "Sir, will I ever fall from the spiritual path?" Yogananda gave a very interesting answer. He replied, "How could you? Everyone in the world is on the spiritual path"—that is to say, not only all human beings, but all animals, all life. God created it all. A woman saint in India, Anandamayee Ma, gave a beautiful answer to somebody who was worried about the direction the world was going. She said, "Don't you think He who made this world knows how to take care of it?" Through people's karma, He'll work things out in His own way, and in His own time.

This universe, the chair that you're sitting on, it seems solid—but it isn't. I hope that I don't talk so long that it seems more solid. The truth is that it's just energy. Scientists themselves are beginning to accept the truth that the Indian sages taught thousands of years ago—that all matter is energy, and that energy is really consciousness. The Infinite Consciousness brought out of itself ideas of what it would create, and then clothed them with will power and energy. Then it vibrated that energy more grossly to become this physical universe. But everything really is God in one form or another—God dreaming, God sleeping in delusion, but nonetheless seeking Itself.

There's an interesting passage in *Autobiography of a Yogi* where Yogananda meets a *gyana* yogi, a follower of the path of discrimination, who has spent his whole life analyzing human motivation. The yogi says that he reached one stark realization: The unifying factor of all mankind is the stalwart kinship of ego motivation. In a way this is so, because we are all motivated by ego, but there's also something higher that unites us.

Yogananda gave a lovely description of God. He said, "The divine vision is center everywhere, circumference nowhere." You are the center of the universe; so am I, and so is everything. The universe is not some big thing imposing itself on a smaller reality. It's created from within each little center radiating outward. In whatever way that you want to explain the universe, you can do so. If you look at it from the standpoint of art, you can understand the entire universe as an expression of aesthetic beauty. If you want to understand it from the perspective of politics, you can see the whole thing in those terms. Wherever you begin, you can understand everything from that point of reference.

All of us have only one point of reference, and that's our own self, our own ego. But Yogananda didn't entirely agree with the gyana yogi because he felt the kinship of all living beings is beyond the ego. There's an aspiration towards something more, towards that which will satisfy the soul. Deep inside each of us there is a yearning for love, joy, and understanding. We think we're going to get these things in human ways by having more money, possessions, or exciting experiences.

In this day and age, our senses are so constantly stimulated that the average human being has an attention span of only one or two seconds. The deeper aspect of it is that we are always dissatisfied with that kind of restlessness. We think that by skating on the surface of life and covering more territory we'll have more experiences, and therefore more wisdom. The fact is we simply become more and more superficial. The more you live at the surface, the further and faster you may be able to skate, but the less you really will absorb or understand.

This point of self-reference, the ego, can go in one of two directions. It can contract inward and think first of "me, me, me." This action makes us more and more a prisoner of littleness and limitation. But there's another direction in which to go—that of the expansive ego. This expression of ego feels other people's sorrow and happiness; it doesn't think in terms of itself alone, but delights in enjoying things through others. The expanded ego finds that in helping and giving to others it becomes freer. But as you follow this line of development, you ultimately realize that there's a limit even to how far this expanded ego can reach out.

I remember many years ago, a friend of mine and I were up on Mt. Waterman in southern California at sunset. It was an extraordinary moment: The sun was setting, the full moon was rising, there was mist in the valleys, and everything was gold and orange. In the opposite direction towards the east, the mist was an ice blue. It was magical! I remember my friend who was really trying to experience it to the fullest finally saying in frustration, "But if only I could *feel* it!" There's a limit to how much you can experience as long as the walls of flesh limit you.

The way to experience that consciousness and beauty everywhere is to rise above body consciousness. This is only done through deep meditation. The more you meditate, the more your senses become refined so that even colors become more beautiful, sounds more entrancing. Everything becomes richer and becomes a part of you. When you can really rise out of body consciousness, suddenly you discover that all this *is* you. You are not just this little ego—you are in all.

I remember Yogananda telling us that once he said to someone, "You have a sour taste in your mouth, don't you?" This person replied in amazement, "How did you know?" Yogananda answered, "Because I'm as much in your body as I am in this body." This is indeed the state of consciousness of a master. There's a story in *Autobiography of a Yogi* in which Lahiri Mahasaya suddenly gasped, "I'm drowning in the bodies of many people in the Sea of Japan." In the newspapers the next day there were headlines about a great disaster at sea off the coast of Japan. Lahiri Mahasaya had felt that. As you approach that expanded state, you begin to become aware of something much more than just a limited egoic experience; you experience the reality of God in everything.

As Master said, "God is center everywhere, circumference nowhere," while the worldly person is circumference everywhere, center nowhere. The average person doesn't think in terms of finding his center—he thinks in terms of seeing things superficially. But all life is a manifestation of one Spirit. Our consciousness can be brought into alignment with that Spirit, so that everything we do will help us to find this inner experience of God.

I've spent nearly fifty years of my life trying to explore this way of looking at life from an inner, central reality. In the books I've written, I try to show how all kinds of different fields which seem very separate—leadership, business, music, the arts, education—are all guided by the same central principles. People may wonder why I write books on so many subjects. The truth is that I write books on only one subject—the underlying central reality of Spirit. I try to show how that subject is pertinent to all these different fields. My hope is that the reader, in understanding what I've done in working from my center, will do the same in his or her life, and do it creatively in a thousand different directions.

When Yogananda came to America, he didn't offer a teaching for only a few people who were really ready. Nor did he offer it only to those few who had had previous spiritual lives in India and managed to slip into an American body this time around. It's true that Master said many Indian souls with spiritual longings are being born into the West. But his purpose was to help all sincere seekers—you, me, all of us—to understand that if we will approach life with this philosophy, and with the practice of Kriya Yoga to magnetize the spine, we will find God. When we do this, and bring all our energy into our inner self, it's amazing how everything in our life falls into place.

I had a very interesting experience many years ago when I was up on the ski slopes. I saw a beginning skier who was bravely trying to make her way down the slope by skiing diagonally, falling, then getting up, and going in the other direction. When instructors try to teach you how to ski, they tell you, "Keep your knees like this, your elbows like that, twist your hips this way, and your poles like that." It's all from the outside. So I said to her, "Something I've found very helpful in skiing is to be centered in your spine. Then you can quickly turn left or right as you need to, and the movements come naturally." I saw her later, and she said, "You know, it works." I watched her, and she was skiing quite well without any sense of tension.

When most people try to learn a new subject, they try to learn it from the outside in. I've seen again and again that the main thing about learning any new subject is persuading yourself that you can do it. Once Yogananda commissioned a well-known artist to do a painting of Lahiri Mahasaya, his guru's guru. When Yogananda saw the painting, he wasn't completely satisfied with it. Though it was technically well done, it didn't capture the consciousness of a spiritual person. He said to the artist, "How long did it take you to master your art?" He replied, "It took me twenty years." Yogananda challenged him by saying, "You mean it took you twenty years to convince yourself you could paint?" Naturally the man got very angry, and said, "I'd like to see you paint as well in twice that length of time!" Yogananda quietly said, "Give me a week." The painter thought that he was being insulted, and turned on his heel.

But Yogananda started. Instead of coming at it from the thought, "I'm not a painter," he tuned in to the consciousness of an artist, and it came naturally. I don't say everyone could do this, but he had that degree of intuition and concentration that made it possible. The first sketch he made didn't work, the next one was better, and by the end of a week he had done a painting that captured the consciousness of Lahiri Mahasaya. Then he had somebody call this artist, and hid himself behind a door. When the artist saw Yogananda's painting, he gasped, "Who did that? It's much better than mine." Yogananda stepped out from behind the door, and said, "You want to know who did it? I did."

There isn't anything that any human being who has ever lived has done that you can't do, if you apply yourself long enough. Yogananda gave us Kriya to show us how to be centered in the spine. From there we can understand how to do anything. We can understand other people and tune in to their consciousness. More than just analyzing them with our minds, we can relate to their center and their reality. I've actually found when checking people's Kriya practice that I can tune in to them and feel when they're doing Kriya properly. How? I get into their center from my own. But you've got to start with a magnetized spine. Then you can really understand other people and perceive solutions to difficulties. You need to look at life in a new way—from your center outward.

Kriya Yoga helps you to develop that vision and ability. Yogananda, in creating a broad base for the pyramid of these teachings, showed us how this central truth can be pertinent to every aspect of life. Whenever you have a problem, get centered in your spine, and a solution will come. I had a wonderful experience in this regard once when I was traveling in India. I had a friend, Dr. Misra, who had lived in California, but had gone back to his native land. Several years later, I went to India and wanted to see him, but I didn't have his address. I knew he lived in Bhubaneswar, which is 200 miles south of Calcutta. I was flying into Calcutta, and thought, "What a pity! I'm coming this close, and still I don't know how to get in touch with him." I landed at the Calcutta airport and was to be met by two friends of mine, but they weren't there. I didn't know what to do or where to go.

The average person would have gotten all upset and rushed to the nearest phone to track people down. It would have been exactly the wrong thing to do. I simply got centered, and inwardly asked, "Well, Divine Mother, what have you got in mind?". Within two seconds somebody who was walking through the airport, and who would have missed me if I'd been dashing off to the telephone, stopped and asked me, "What is your good name?" This is the way they express themselves in India. I've always liked that presumption that it's a good name.

I told him, and he said, "Ah, I thought it must be you. A friend of mine, Dr. Misra, showed me a photograph of you, and I've been longing to meet you." I said, "Dr. Misra? This is the very person I've been wanting to meet! Can you give me his address in Bhubaneswar?" He said happily, "Oh, you don't have to go to Bhubaneswar. I've just come to Calcutta myself to meet him. He happens to be staying here." So he took me to his home. A further interesting thing was that all the hotels in Calcutta on that particular evening were full, and I wouldn't have had a place to stay. As it turned out, I had a home to stay in and a wonderful visit with my friend.

I've seen this kind of thing happen again and again, if you resist the usual human tendency to try to solve problems from the outside rather than being centered and letting the universe help you. You find that somehow with inward peace and harmony, everything seems to go well. This also applies to what you need to learn and what you have to study.

In *Autobiography of a Yogi* Yogananda tells the story about how he didn't really want to study for his college exams. He had been spending all his time with his guru, not in the classroom, but because he was doing a spiritual thing, somehow he passed those exams without studying. Now I'm not offering this as guidance to any of you of school age, but if you put God first, things somehow work out. In the *Bhagavad Gita* it says, "Know this for a certainty, Arjuna: My devotee is never lost." God may give you big tests, and they may seem terrible at the time. We read the story of Job and of other devotees who were tested because of their faith and devotion in order to set an example for others. But if you really hang in there, you win in the end. Sometimes it's an end that's around the corner, or even around several corners, but ultimately faith in God wins out.

I had a fascinating experience before I met Master which shows that any of us can work with these principles on our own level. I was in college at the time, though I wasn't learning much because the classes were too intellectual without any heart quality. I was taking a course in Greek, but didn't study and rarely came to class. Toward the end of the semester when I would be called on to translate from Greek into English, I would be so at sea that it was an embarrassment. The professor would say, "There are some people who might as well not come to the final exam," and everybody would look at me and laugh. But something in me was determined and said, "I'm going to pass this exam."

So a week before the final, I picked up the Greek text and tried to read a little bit, but just put it down. It was totally incomprehensible. I thought, "I'll study twice as long tomorrow." Famous last words. The next night I didn't study, nor the next, until finally the night before the exam, I realized I hadn't studied at all. Still, for some crazy reason, I was absolutely sure that I would pass. In that crisis, I came upon a great discovery. Instead of thinking, "I've got to learn Greek, though it's absolutely foreign to me," I just told myself, "You *are* a Greek."

I picked up the book and, in some subtle and strange way, I began absorbing the language like my own. When you put yourself in tune with something, there is a subtle network that ties us all together. I didn't know what I was doing, but even in my lack of knowledge, I hit upon the principle of approaching the subject from the inside out. I read the Greek book with great concentration. There was none of this pulling toward me with part of my mind and pushing away with the other, which is usually the way we study. If you push on opposite sides of a door, you can exhaust yourself, but the door doesn't move. Because all my will and energy were moving in the same direction, suddenly I was absorbing Greek as though my mind were a sponge.

Another very interesting thing happened that night as I was preparing for the exam. We'd been studying the New Testament in Greek and were going to have to translate one chapter on the test. I thought, "I only have time to read one chapter in English, but if I have the right consciousness that will be the chapter on the exam." And it was. Since I had read this chapter in English, I knew what it was all about. There were only two people in the class who passed the exam, and I was one of them. Later the professor said, "You really studied, didn't you?" I didn't dare answer!

But in fact I did study, because there was no struggle to learn. I just absorbed the language because I convinced myself I was a Greek. Whatever you do, the main thing is to persuade yourself you can succeed by starting at the center of it. You'll find that suddenly you're in tune, and it will come naturally.

With this understanding, Yogananda brought Kriya Yoga, not only as a means of finding success in what you do, but of finding divine enlightenment. This indeed is what all of life is about. This is the thing that binds us all together, even with our differences. There is that hunger in each of us for the divine state. We mistake it for so many things, for this desire or that yearning, that it can take us millions of lifetimes to get out of delusion. As Yogananda said in his interpretations of the *Rubaiyat of Omar Khayyam,* "Many people are still wandering in delusion who were here in physical bodies at the dawn of this day of Brahma." Who knows how many billions of years this has been? Will we still be wandering in delusion at the end of this day of Brahma? It's a frightening thought.

But you can see why it takes so long when you when you think of how many mistakes people can make. How many times do they think, "Oh, this is my answer," or, "That's my answer"? All the time they don't realize that they're just picking up shiny bits of broken glass from the ground and thinking that they're diamonds. But it's just glass all the same. Everything in this world that you think will make you happy never does. If it does for a while, it won't for very long. Nothing brings us lasting happiness—absolutely nothing. Only one thing will truly satisfy you, and that's to know the inner peace of your own self.

As St. Augustine said, "Lord, thou hast made us for Thyself alone, and our hearts are restless until they find their rest in Thee." This is the truth of it—you will never find what you're looking for until you become That yourself. It isn't in bank accounts or in beautiful paintings. The longer you go on this path, the more you begin to realize none of the things you've been seeking have brought you the answer.

So Kriya Yoga is that all-important key which, metaphorically speaking, helps to align your molecules, your inner flow of consciousness, in a unified direction so that your bar of steel, your spine, becomes a magnet. When all your energy is going in one direction, the little contrary pulls of the ego have no power. It takes a lot of effort to accomplish this, but it's worth it. In fact it's the only thing that is worth it because ultimately it's the only thing that works at all. Once you've done that, suddenly you find that you're at home wherever you go.

There's a lovely story of a saint from India called Ram Tirtha who came to the West around the turn of the century. He felt the inspiration to come here, and though he hadn't any money and didn't know anyone, somehow he got a boat passage to America. He was on the boat coming into San Francisco harbor, when a man standing next to him on the deck asked him, "Is someone meeting you here?" "No," he said. Again the man asked, "Do you know anything about this country?" "No," Ram Tirtha said cheerfully. The surprised man continued, "Do you have friends in this country?" "I have one," he replied happily. "Well, who is it?" the man asked. "You." This man, who happened to be quite wealthy, was so charmed by this answer that he sponsored Ram Tirtha's lecture tour around the country.

You'll be surprised how wonderfully things work if you don't run around frantically, but just get centered in yourself. Then you're at home wherever you go, and everybody is your friend. Even your enemies are your friends because they're helping you in some way, though they may not know it. It's not as if they help you consciously, but the Divine gives you whatever experiences you need in order to find your own self and to discover that your true self is one with the Infinite. You are sons and daughters of the Infinite Consciousness. You were born for that, and you will never be happy until you've found that.

In bringing Kriya Yoga to the West, Yogananda did something that most great saints have not done. Usually they tell you, "The world is all delusion. Meditate and leave it all behind." Yogananda took more the approach of the Vedas. He showed that by using Kriya you can change yourself, and from your spiritual center you can help transform this world. It's an important lesson, because if the world is totally uninvolved in anything spiritual, then the devotee is isolated and alone without any support for his aspirations. But Yogananda saw that if he could transform an entire civilization, even to some extent, then the whole civilization would support the deeper spiritual search of the few. He went out from that center of Kriya Yoga and showed how relevant it is to all walks of life.

Indeed, he came to usher in what they call in India a new *Yuga*, a new age. We're only at the very beginning of his mission, but if you want to see what changes that mission will bring, stick around for a few hundred years. You'll see how it will transform all society, because it will help people who don't know where they're going suddenly to understand. Our whole civilization is teetering on the brink of chaos, yet it will be transformed by this simple but universal truth. I think, for this reason, we're living in one of the most exciting times possible—a time when the whole human race, not quickly but slowly and ineluctably, will be transformed from the inside out.

The science of Kriya Yoga has value beyond measure because it helps you to become centered so that everything you do somehow improves. It proceeds from your center into attunement with that Divine Consciousness, which is center everywhere, circumference nowhere.

Do any of you have questions?

Q: *If you are sensitive to negativity in other people, and you're in a situation where you can't avoid them, what can you do?*

A: I'm glad you asked that question because it's a very important one. If you're sensitive to negative vibrations, you must use your superconsciousness which is solution-oriented to find the way out. Your sensitivity can actually be useful in this way. I had a very interesting experience once in Rome when I was having dinner with an acquaintance and his wife. A friend of mine, who was also present, said afterwards, "My God, the negativity those people have!" I was surprised that he was so sensitive to their negativity and thought, "Really? I didn't notice anything." Then suddenly I realized that my entire evening had been spent trying to give them suggestions that might help them to get out of those problems. I wasn't thinking of the negativity, but rather of solutions that would help.

In this way you can be sensitive but use that sensitivity to help others rather than be drawn down by their negativity. Try to think in terms of what you can give people, of letting God tell you how to help them. Then you will find great blessings even in sorrow, because nothing is inherently negative or bad. It's all neutral, but it seems good or bad depending on the way you look at it.

If you see someone who's deformed, and you're thinking in terms of helping him or her, you see only beauty because you see underneath the deformity the hunger of the soul to come out. In any problem or negativity that we face in life, there's something inside that wants something better. If you tune in to that underlying yearning, then you'll find that it's possible to help. So it's very important not to get sucked into negativity, but to use your sensitivity to find the opposing quality or energy that can cure the problem. Does that help?

Q: *I think so, but what if you're in a situation that's really overwhelming where you can't think of anything to do?*

A: Those situations definitely occur where you feel that you can't help. What do you do? You simply have to give it to God. When you go to a poor country and see hundreds of beggars, if you give money to one, soon you'll be mobbed by a crowd. What do you do about it? You can only bless them. You can help a few, but you can't help everybody. If you were a millionaire and gave one dollar to a million people, which is a small percentage of the world anyway, what good would it really do them? It would be far better to use that money to build a hospital. In other words, it's better to do something that would reach many more people in a qualitative way.

The main thing is we have to remain channels of light and try to serve in that way. Basically there's very little we can do anyway to help in an outward way. In building Ananda, if people came to me with too many problems, or even too many objections to a particular idea, I would say, "I don't want to hear about it. We won't draw the right answers or directions by focusing on the problems." If my mind slips out of the creative flow, I can't draw solutions.

We need to maintain that attitude which will keep us creative, charitable, and positive. It you're seeing too much negativity, then just close the door, because there's a limit to what one person, or even many people, can do. Keep as your priority to have an uplifted consciousness first. If you don't have money in the bank, you can't give it to help others. If you don't have strength, you can't give it to anybody. You have to give of your riches—you can't give of your poverty. Your first responsibility is to be in tune, and from that attunement do what you can. But don't get frantic, and don't allow negativity to pull you down. Best of all, do what you can with a sense of joy, freedom, and love.

Q: *They say that consciousness continues after you die. I was wondering, are you able to communicate with your master through your meditation?*

A: I don't like to talk about myself much, but I will say something about this because I think it's important. Master's reality to me now isn't the things that he did or said. Those are manifestations of that reality, but they're not the essence of his reality. More and more I find that if I tune in to him about something I'm doing—my music or writing—or if I'm trying to find a new direction in life, I feel his consciousness and in that I feel the inspiration of how to proceed. Then from that inspiration stories spontaneously come into my mind—memories of things he said or did—to corroborate that inspiration.

At that point I deliberately try to think of anything he might have said or done that would contradict that inspiration, because the mind can fool itself. I don't trust this mind for a moment. So I try to shoot it down with other recollections, but I let them come in later because that's the negative side. The critical intellect is not creative, but it's a very important part of our mental baggage. You need it to discriminate and say, "Am I kidding myself, or is it really so?" If I can't think of anything that contradicts it, and if I still feel this inspiration, then I go with it. I find that this works. So, yes, I do feel his presence, and this is how I use it in what I do.

Q: *Should I pray to God for specific things or just for God's guidance to show me what to do?*

A: There's an amusing story that a friend of mine in Australia told me about a man who died and went to heaven. St. Peter showed him around, and finally he was shown the heavenly junkyard. This was the place where they collected all the things that people had rejected while on earth. The man said, "That's absurd. Who would turn down that Cadillac over there?" St. Peter said, "It's interesting that you should ask that question because, in fact, you're the person who turned it down." The man said, "That's ridiculous. I never turned down a Cadillac." St. Peter said, "Oh, yes, you did. Every time you prayed for a car, you visualized a Volkswagen."

God has greater things in store for us than we know. If we're too specific in our requests, we often find that we don't get the best thing for us. In fact, we often get the worst because we didn't know that it wasn't right for us. So it's good to pray for things, but best of all is to offer everything to God and say, "You choose what's best for me." You'll find He chooses better than you would. He's also got a great sense of humor. Often God gives you exactly the thing you didn't want, but if you go with faith you find that it was the only thing that ever could have worked.

Chapter Five

Paramhansa Yogananda—
The Power of Divine Love

"You can only understand another human being if you approach him with deep compassion and love."

I'd like to pay homage to the life of one of God's children—an enlightened being with the humility of a child who was one we call "Master." We use this word not in the sense of our being his servants, but because he was master of himself. Through his example, he can also help us to become masters of ourselves, of our passions and lower nature, in order to discover who we really are. Our goal in life, whether we know it or not, is to fulfill our potential as human beings.

There's a story of a woman saint in Kashmir, India who used to wear no clothing because she had renounced everything. A scandalized villager once said to her, "Why don't you wear any clothes?" She answered, "Why should I? I see no men around." To her rather drastic view, nobody even deserved to be called a human being so long as his or her consciousness was still on the physical plane. Then one day a saint came to visit her, and as soon as she learned he'd arrived, she began rushing around looking for clothing to wear. She explained, "Finally a man has come," and she had to be modest before him.

This slightly unconventional way of looking at things is nonetheless the attitude of divine beings who look around and see that most people aren't really much above dogs and cats. We have a little more intelligence, but we're still running around in circles, as kittens do, chasing our tails or little puffs of wool. Most people don't yet know what life is all about.

One of the things that Yogananda brought to us was the understanding of the real secret of life. There was a very funny cartoon by George Price of a woman in the kitchen of a tenement flat with plaster cracking off the walls, and with children tugging at her skirts in opposite directions. She's trying to do the ironing, and her husband is sitting on the windowsill in his undershirt playing the tuba. The caption underneath says, "Can't you play anything except 'Ah, Sweet Mystery of Life'?" In that song, love is the "mystery of life."

Most people don't understand what love really means, or how deeply fulfilling it is. I'm not speaking of love for a person, but of love itself, love for God. It's not a sweet sentiment or a feeling that makes you weepy—it's something incredibly powerful. I remember once standing in the doorway saying goodbye to Yogananda, and he looked at me with a power that was overwhelming. I'm near-sighted, so it wasn't his expression that I saw, but it was a power that came out of his eyes and overwhelmed me. I stood rooted to the spot. The kind of power that he brought is what this world needs today.

I had an interesting experience many years ago when I was in Self-Realization Fellowship. At that time I used to review exams from students of the lessons to see if they'd understood the material. Usually the answers they sent were pretty standard, within a narrow range of response, and I could quickly see whether they'd read the right passage or not. But it was strange, because every now and then, some very unusual answer would be sent in. Within a few weeks this would happen several times, and I would get the same answer from all over the world—Australia, Germany, Italy, and Africa. After this flurry of letters with the unusual answer, it would never happen again. I began to think, "My goodness, there's literal truth to what Yogananda wrote in *Autobiography of a Yogi,* when he said, 'Thoughts are universally, not individually, rooted.'"

A man can perceive a truth; he can't create it. Somebody asked me yesterday, "I want to be creative. How can I learn to do something original that nobody else has ever done?" I said, "Original means to come from your own point of origin. It doesn't mean doing something no one else has done, but doing something that is completely true to you." Think of something common like the simple phrase "I love you." How many millions of times has that phrase been uttered? Many times, though certainly not always, it has very deep meaning because it's sincere.

I also mentioned to him the example of Beethoven's Seventh Symphony with that beautiful Second Movement which is fundamentally so simple. If Beethoven proposed it to you, and said, "Hey, I've got this hot idea for a tune," and sang it, you'd have said, "It won't work. It won't sell. They won't like it on Broadway." The chords themselves are the most basic ones you use when you're harmonizing—the tonic, dominant, and subdominant—and yet it's one of the loveliest pieces of music ever written. Why? Because he felt it! And when you feel a thing deeply within it's going to express that power.

Anything you do sincerely, from your own source within, cannot but be different from whatever has been done before because you are unique. No one will ever be you. No one will ever be able to sing the song that the Infinite has given you to sing. Each thumbprint is unique, and how much more so is each individual consciousness. In the Indian scriptures they say that every atom is endowed with individuality. This individuality is an aspect of Spirit manifesting in nature, and it's an aspect of who you really are.

When a great master comes into this world, he comes to show us not who *he* is, but who *we* are. In trying to find who we are, it also helps us to understand who we aren't. Most of our self-definitions are false because they're based on externals. You aren't a man or a woman, for starters. These are just bodies we put on for a while, because our hormones influence us in certain ways. This is what causes a woman to act like a woman, and a man like a man. There was an interesting case of a male novelist who underwent a sex change operation. He, along with all his readers, noticed that after the operation he wrote completely differently, with a much more feminine consciousness.

Our hormones definitely have an influence over us, but ultimately we are souls which are neither male nor female. You think, "I'm an American," or "I'm a Japanese," but this is just an act that you've assumed. When you were born, you were brought up in this country, and so you act like an American. I was born in Rumania of American parents, so it was very difficult for me after coming to this country to try to adjust to the American way of looking at things. It took me a long time to be able to work with Americans and help them understand these teachings, and in a way I'm still learning. But it's been helpful because it's forced me to become more aware of the process of "Americanization," and not just take it for granted.

However, I know that's not who I am. That's not who you are—you're something far more. In fact it's interesting to see how thoughts sweep the world, just as with those people who sent in the unusual answers for the exams I mentioned earlier. We find fads sweeping the world, and suddenly everybody's playing with the hula hoop, or listening to a new kind of music. Suddenly everybody is all for, or all against, Clinton. You go through enough decades of this, and you see that it's all just nothing. I never watch television, read newspapers, or listen to the radio anymore. People ask me, "How do you keep up with news?" I answer them, "If there's anything of importance that happens, people will tell me." I just don't find it interesting because it all seems like gossip.

The reality of who you are is something far deeper. When you live in that reality, you begin to feel these deeper currents of consciousness. Each one of us is an example of the inner soul that's at the center of life, striving to come out and discover who it really is. In a way, the life of any individual is the life of all individuals.

When I wrote my book, *The Path*, at first I thought, "I'll never be able to really reach people in a meaningful way because my life has been so different." Not many people are born outside their own country, or have had all the experiences that happened in my youth. But the most common reaction that I've received in letters from people who've read *The Path* has been, "I felt that you were describing my life." I'm very grateful, because that's what I'd hoped. If, however, this is true, then I'm sorry for everybody because my life initially was so confused. I had it completely backwards.

I wanted to know what truth was, and in my effort to find it, I read a lot and developed all sorts of theories. I tried to find out what the meaning of life was through science, politics, art, literature, music, and all sorts of intellectual means. Finally I began to realize that I was walking through a desert—it was all mental, intellectual, and empty. I began to remember my childhood, and how happy I'd been when I'd been living more in the heart.

Finally I got fed up with how intellectual I was, and realized that every time I tried to change one aspect of myself, a problem would pop up in another area. It was like washing a shirt—you try to submerge all of it under water, but a bubble of air comes up under one part and pushes the shirt up there. So you try to push that bubble down, and another bubble comes up in a different place. No matter where you push the shirt down, a bubble comes up somewhere else. In every way that I tried to change myself, and I tried many ways, I found I was just going around in circles like a dance—forward, backward, forward, backward. I realized that I didn't have the understanding to know what I really needed to do. I was like Ogden Nash's poem about the llama: "This poor benighted have not / Don't even know what he ain't got."

I remember, however, there was one thought that was very strong in me. I felt that there had to be some kind of consciousness behind it all, some kind of God. But to me at that time, God was just an abstraction. Then when I read *Autobiography of a Yogi,* I was so absolutely moved between laughter and tears, between the greatest joy I'd ever known and tears of even greater joy. I took the next bus across America and came to Los Angeles to meet him. Through him, I discovered that the real meaning to life is indeed just like in that song, "Ah, Sweet Mystery of Life." It is love. When you can love, you have everything—and when your heart is closed, you have nothing.

Yogananda's way of loving was very different from what you might think. It was not a sweet sentiment or a gentle expression. It was that kind of power that could oppose evil, but with love and respect. Sometimes he scolded us because he was trying to get a thought into our minds to help us understand it properly. At such times I would look into his eyes and see a deep regret that he had to talk to us so strongly. He didn't enjoy scolding, but even when he did it, he never got angry. You could feel that he had enough love to be able to stand up and attack our delusions head on, and to tell us what we needed to hear.

It wasn't as though if you'd murdered your mother, and asked him, "Did I do something wrong?" he'd say, "Well, everybody's got his problems." No, he'd tell you, "You did wrong." Why did you do wrong? It's not because there's a law in this country against murder, or because there's a chance that you might go to prison and get executed. You did wrong primarily against your own soul, against yourself.

Master had that kind of power and wisdom in his love that was always working for your true welfare, though living with him was definitely not a mutual admiration society. True, we had plenty of admiration for him, and he had infinite admiration for our soul capacity. But he certainly didn't admire our delusions, or even what we considered our virtues. To him they were nothing.

I remember telling him once about some spiritual experience I was having. To take me off my high horse, he just said, "That's nothing." The real power in his life was that he loved God in you. He was not the friend of your ego. He was the friend of God in you, and that divine spark which, whether you know it or not, always longs to escape from limitation and discover its oneness with the Infinite.

Sometimes he encountered quite serious situations because of his uncompromising dedication to truth. There was a marvelous story about him that occurred many years ago during the Depression. He had given a talk saying that it is wrong for rich people to take advantage of the poor. He said it was a tremendous injustice to make them even poorer in order to become richer, and he even named a few names of wealthy people who had done this. Afterwards his friends told him, "You'd better not go home alone tonight," but he said, "I'm not afraid. God is with me." Sure enough as he came to a dark section of the town before entering the train station to go home, a man came up behind him and put a pistol in his back. The gunman said, "Why did you talk that way about those people?" Completely fearlessly, Yogananda said, "All people are God's children. God isn't pleased when His rich children take advantage of His poor children." Imagine talking like this to someone who's got a contract to kill you. Then he turned around and looked into this man's eyes with great love—not the kind of love that is approving, but the kind that sears your ego down to ashes. Holding him in the power of his love, Yogananda said, "Why do you live the way you do? You aren't happy. I demand that Satan come out of you!" The man began to tremble all over, and finally he said, "What have you done to me? I was sent to kill you, but I can't go back to that way of living anymore." The man's life was completely changed.

That kind of power is what he brought. It isn't just a lovely teaching, but something that is life shattering. People read *Autobiography of a Yogi,* and they get the impression that he was so soft, loving, and sweet. Indeed he was all of those qualities, no doubt about it, but he was also extremely powerful. When people listen to his voice on tape recordings that he made, they are invariably shocked because he talked with so much power. His voice thunders out, "I, Paramhansa Yogananda, am praying with you."

I remember the lecture he gave in Beverly Hills, which I've mentioned in *The Path,* where he was rallying people to go out and start communities everywhere. He said, "Youths, go North, South, East, and West. . . ." It wasn't as if he were shouting, but I could feel this power surging through him. He was not even he. He was a wave of that Infinite Consciousness which comes and spreads out on the shore, like waves rushing up onto the beach through rocks; they break up into little streamlets, and then withdraw again.

So that Divine Consciousness comes into this world and breaks up into all sorts of different attitudes and outlooks. Whether you know it or not, you are the product of those diverse attitudes. You are not your personality. It is just an aggregate of all the things you've done and the reactions you've had. The true you is behind all of that. When you come to understand this, then you see that Yogananda, too, was not as he appeared. He said, "I killed Yogananda long ago. No one dwells in this temple now but God." He was a manifestation without any ego, without any sense of "I like this," or "I want that." To him, it was all the Divine. When I looked into his eyes, it was in a very real way like looking into infinity.

Different saints come on earth with different missions. In one way or another, all of them have love, but they don't always show it because that may not be their mission. It *was* Yogananda's mission to express divine love, and because of that he talked of God in a new way—one that we're not used to in this country. He spoke of God as the Divine Mother. Now, in truth, God is neither mother nor father, but He's that Absolute Consciousness beyond creation. However, God does manifest Himself in different ways, so you can say that God is also both father and mother.

He's unique to each one of us because as we visualize Him, so He will come in the form we hold most dear. If we happen to have some special and unusual reverence for crocodiles, and worship God as a Divine Crocodile, that's how He will come to us. But, of course, that's not necessarily inspiring to most people , whereas the mother aspect of God is something that satisfies a deep longing in the heart.

When we think of God, we're just not satisfied with the image of a judge or with dry intellectual definitions. The more male aspect is a very important component of humanity, and we certainly wouldn't be able to function without it. When I read in *Time* magazine that the extreme feminists are putting down men to such a great extent, I can't help thinking that that's like one side of a coin accusing the other of being made of debased metal. It's ridiculous, because we're all the same species.

There are two aspects to human nature—reason and feeling. Science has taught us, and unfortunately we've bought the lie, that the only way to come to truth is to exclude feeling and be so objective that you're only intellectual. The truth is that if you get to know any really great scientists, even through their life stories, you find that they were passionate men and women. They were absolutely dedicated to the search for scientific truth. Nor could they have accomplished what they did without deep feeling and enthusiasm for what they were doing. It has been said that no great thing has ever been accomplished without enthusiasm.

Thomas Edison, for example, went through forty-three thousand experiments before he found the right filament for the light bulb. His own co-workers were pleading with him to stop when he reached twenty thousand attempts, but he was sure that a solution had to be there. It was the heart quality that led him forward. It's only the second-rate scientists who do petty little experiments that go exclusively by intellect, but real scientists are people of deep mystical awe before the wonders of the universe. Awe is expressed in their experiments and their theories. Without that sense of wonder, how could they have discovered the great things they've found?

This enthusiasm is a part of the heart quality. We, as human beings, have both heart and intellect, but we can never reach true understanding with only the intellect. The thought that you can mentally analyze people, and therefore understand them, is a fallacy. You can only understand another human being if you approach him with deep compassion and love. You can only understand yourself with love for yourself, not for your faults, but for your real nature. You'll never find understanding if you just look at yourself analytically, which usually includes judgment—that won't give it to you. But try to love your own potential, to have respect for who you are as a child of God. This is also a part of the heart quality.

Both that love which unites and the intellect which separates are necessary. But until you can feel your kinship with all life, and understand others from within, you won't know their true reality. Try to understand why others do what they do, even when they're doing wrong things, or are trying to hurt you. Try to understand where they're coming from, and you'll be amazed at how much compassion that gives you.

In our culture today, this heart quality has been gradually seeping into the sands and disappearing, until we find ourselves in an age which emphasizes only analysis, intellect, and mental definitions. As a result, although we think we understand, somehow we always seem to be just one step away from real truth and understanding. No matter how cleverly we analyze, we're still just that far from really knowing.

There's a beautiful story of Krishna as a little boy that illustrates this principle. He was being very mischievous, so his foster mother decided to tie him to a bedpost. She took a string and tied him up, but the string was a little too short to tie him up properly. She got another string and tied it to the first so that it was more than long enough. But somehow when she'd finished, it was still a little bit too short. No matter how much string she added, it still remained too short.

Of course the moral of the story is that you cannot bind the Infinite. But you can also apply this moral when it comes to trying to understand the Infinite with just your own mind. Without that element of intuition, without that element of feeling and love, you can't really understand anything. You can't bind any reality of life with a definition. Yes, you can get an airplane off the ground. Yes, you can figure out how many miles it is from here to the sun, but what does it really matter?

To understand how to live your life better, to understand other people, and to understand truth, you can't do it without heart. To think of God as the mother aspect is a way of helping you to love from your heart and to approach God in an infinite way. Yogananda used to say, "Mother, naughty or good, I am Your child." In India they say that bad sons there are many, but never has there been a bad mother. I've heard many Indians say this sentimentally as a human truth, but the unfortunate fact is that there have been many bad mothers. But there can never be a bad Divine Mother, because she is your own true friend, your highest friend.

So Yogananda brought to this country one of the most important spiritual gifts possible—the idea of worshiping the Divine Mother. I was meditating in Italy a year and a half ago, and the thought came to me that we need to especially emphasize this aspect of his teachings: the aspect of deep, personal love for God, for the Divine Mother. The qualities of compassion and of yearning are what will bring you to God.

You could live next door to the best restaurant. You could know everything on their menu, but if you aren't hungry, you aren't going to go there and eat. Hunger is what's needed to make you act. The hunger for God is what's needed to make you decide, "Yes, I want to give my life for this," not, "Yeah, it's a good idea, and I'm sure glad somebody else is doing it." You need that hunger yourself.

There's a story of a boy who came to a saint and asked to become his disciple. The saint said, "Come with me," and he took him down to the river. The saint held the boy's head under the water, until the boy began kicking furiously. Still the saint held him under, so that he was struggling with all his strength to break free. Finally he let him up. Then he said to the boy, "What did you want most when your head was under water?" The gasping boy replied, "AAir, AAAir!!!" The saint said, "When you want God as much as you wanted air, come back, and I'll accept you as my disciple."

We have to long for God. We have to reach that point where nothing means anything except that. That's why the best thing you can pray for is devotion—the ability to love God more and more deeply. Yogananda came to bring us that. Remember that no matter what you do, God's on your side. He's not going to judge you—he's going to help you in every way He can, but you have to let Him help you. On the other hand, He'll make you work for it. Even salvation is nothing without the love of God. If you achieve it, perhaps you go to another plane where you don't have to eat food, or carry around a heavy body, but there still are problems. Without God, you've got problems, let's face it. He's the only solution. It will get pretty boring even in heaven until you know what it's really all about.

Think of God as the nearest of the near, the dearest of the dear. Women owe it to themselves and to the human race to bring out that loving and understanding aspect of their nature, just as men owe it to the human race to be wise and emotionally balanced in their thinking. When women today feel the need to be heard, they're really responding to a current in the Divine Consciousness that is asking the human race to become balanced. Women who try to be like men are missing the point. When either men or women become out of balance in their nature, they become full of flaws—men become cold and hard, and women become overly emotional. Neither is good, yet both sides have a special gift to give others.

Ultimately, we all need to rise above thinking of ourselves as men or women, so that we can find that perfect balance where Divine Consciousness lies. Yogananda was a beautiful combination of masculine and feminine qualities. Anandamayee Ma, a great woman saint that I knew in India, was in many ways like a man—not in a human way, but in the sense of having reason and feeling well balanced. Whenever she answered questions, it was in such an abstract way that it was sometimes quite astonishing. Her definition of God was, "It is, and It isn't, and neither is It, nor is It not." You make something of that one! You'd expect that a male devotee would be more likely to be impersonal, but male saints often become more feminine, in the sense of being very tender, generous, and kind. The two together show what we should be as human beings.

Men saints even develop breasts a little bit. Look at Lahiri Mahasaya's picture.* They develop the heart quality so much that it manifests itself physically to some extent with a softened chest. Men who are overly intellectual and lacking feeling usually have a narrow, caved-in chest because there's no energy there. It's all going up to the brain. So when you have a balanced nature, you find that your very body expresses it.

Women become much more decisive in their behavior and in their way of moving and walking. Anandamayee Ma would sometimes look like a general walking, and yet she also had a motherly, loving quality that was captivating. I'm Master's disciple, and I've never thought of changing my discipleship, but I had the opportunity to be with her, and it was wonderful. I remember the last time I saw her. I was leaving for the train station, and she said goodbye, but I just stood there. She said goodbye again, and still I just stood fixed to the spot. Finally I said, "Mother, I can't move until you leave." Then she smiled and went inside, and then I was free to go. I just couldn't move until she left, because that love was some-

*Editor's note: He is Yogananda's guru's guru, and his life is described in *Autobiography of a Yogi*.

thing so real and tangible that nothing else had any meaning or reality.

I used to look at some of her disciples who would be running after her to see what she said or did, or to whom she was talking. To me, her reality, and Master's reality as well, was best felt sitting in the back of the room and trying to feel their vibration and love pouring over me. Once you feel it, you think, "There's nothing else that matters. Nothing."

You could die, or suffer a terrible disease, or lose all your material goods, but the only thing that matters is that love. When you have it, everything seems to go smoothly. I've seen again and again that this love is a reality that also manifests itself in the practical world. If I lose that, no matter what I do to make things work, they don't go properly.

Recently I was in Rishikesh, India where I was meditating and having a period of seclusion. It was a strange time, however. Many people doubt, or even flatly deny, the existence of Satan, but all saints have said that Satan is a reality. He's not somebody with a red suit and a long tail , but it's a consciousness that tries to keep everything in delusion. Anybody who's tried to combat delusion has found that he's got a fight on his hands. In Rishikesh, for some reason, that force was trying to attack me. Almost every day I would find a great sense of negativity come upon me. It wasn't that I was being negative, but a thought force would come upon me saying, "It's no use. Why even try spiritually?" It was trying to make me feel discouraged, pessimistic, and to bring my consciousness down. I would try to reason through it, and to fight against it, but nothing worked. Finally I found the one thing that did work—just attuning myself to my Guru. As soon as I just offered it up to him, in a split second it vanished, and I would suddenly feel as if the blue sky had returned.

It was as if the sunshine burst through the clouds, and I felt completely free. Then the next day there was the same struggle, and again the same solution. But I found that everyday I was feeling more and more joy, until at the end this period, I was just floating in joy.

Don't worry about the tests and negativity when they come to you, and don't try to reason your way out of them, because you won't be able to. Ultimately reason will just take you in circles. Give yourself to the Divine Mother, to the Guru, to God in any form that attracts you. From your heart, say, "I am yours," and you will see that, again and again, the darkness will vanish. In fact, it will turn out to have been intended as a blessing all along. It will be a blessing, but it has to be first understood as a grace, so that you don't become angry or bitter.

I get so sad when I see this country going more and more toward anger and bitterness, with everybody wanting to sue somebody else. This victim consciousness that says, "I'm this way because people did this to me," is so wrong. You're this way because *you* made yourself that way—if not in this life, then in another, but you invited it. What will strengthen you is not getting rid of the person or the problem, but changing yourself. When you can become strong enough in yourself, suddenly you'll find that what happens doesn't really touch you. People can say all manner of things against you, and you'll just take it with good humor because you see that it doesn't matter.

There are certain attitudes that come with grace, and this inner strength is one of them. But another is to live for the Divine Mother and to see Her everywhere—not as a person with a form, but as a consciousness in everything. Think of God behind the rocks and clouds. Think that God is saying something to you personally, and you'll see that bit by bit, your relationship with Him really will be personal. It could be that way right now if we could open up to that love. Granted that He's infinite and impersonal, but you are one of His unique creations, and He can relate to you according to your understanding. If you will open your mind and heart to Him, you'll see that you can have a very intimate rapport with Him that becomes sweet beyond anything you can imagine.

I remember when I was in the Porziuncola in Assisi, Italy, where St. Francis died. I prayed to St. Francis, and all of a sudden I felt this intense sweetness come over me. I had never imagined that human nature could be so sweet, and I said, "Please tell me, how is it possible to have such sweetness?" The answer that was given to me was, "By never judging another human being, by seeing all as your brothers and sisters, by accepting them all as your own, by being humble, but above all, by never judging." Then I felt that sweetness so strongly that I was floating on a cloud of sweetness for the rest of the day. How wonderful life is when your heart begins to flower.

There's a lovely song of Ram Proshad, one of the great saints of Bengal, that says, "Your eyes will flow with tears just singing 'God, God, God.' A thousand Vedas tell us that my Divine Mother is without form." He is saying that a true devotee of Kali, or Divine Mother, does not really worship Her in form, but sees Her everywhere. There is another lovely story, which I've mentioned in *The Path*, about the saint Namdev, who found enlightenment when he reached the point where he saw God, not only in the temple, but everywhere.

We need to strive to achieve that state of consciousness so that everywhere we look, we see God, we see the Divine Mother. You can experience this if you get away from singing *about* Him, which is always in the third person, and start thinking more in terms of singing *to* Him. Talk to God. Share every thought with Him. Here's a very interesting experiment to try. Start tonight, try it for a few days, and see if it doesn't change your consciousness. Talk to God in the second person. Say, "God, where do you want me to go today? God, what do you want me to eat today?" These may seem like trivial things, but to Him nothing's trivial. What you eat, or whom you see is just as important to Him as asking, "What great mission shall I accomplish?" The really important thing is that you include Divine Mother in your thoughts and in your heart. Share every thought, every impression, every feeling with Her. Then you will see that in a very short time, there comes into your life a divine symphony, and you'll be floating on clouds of joy.

This was perhaps the main thing that Yogananda came to bring to the world. It isn't that other saints haven't talked of the need to love God. But he did it in a unique and particularly strong way because he did it with great power. When you feel the power of that love, it's shattering. I'll be honest with you because I don't want to trick you—that love will shatter all your false preconceptions of what life's all about. It will show you that life is altogether different from what you thought it was, and that all the things that you thought were so important aren't at all. They're just dust.

In contrast, many of the things that you thought were unimportant turn out to be the most important things of all. Let's say, for example, that you are on your way to a big business conference where you have to sign an important contract. On the way, you meet a beggar and give him a little money. Perhaps you think, "Well, that was nothing. Signing that big contract is the important thing." Later you wake up and realize, "No, giving the money to the beggar was the important thing because it was a little manifestation of divine love." The love that you express for other people is more important than anything else you do. The kindness that you express, the humility in embracing their needs along with your own, and above all, doing it in God's name—these are the things that give life value.

I met a man while traveling once who gave me a hard-luck story and asked for money. I didn't know if his sob story was genuine, but I gave him most of the money I had in my wallet. Later it turned out not to be true, but at the time I felt if I didn't give him the money, and he was genuinely in need, I would feel badly. As I gave him the money, he said to me, "I'll be sure you get it back, because I don't want you to lose faith in human nature." I said, "Listen, if I had faith in human nature, I'd have lost it a long time ago. I have faith in God. I'm not giving this to you, I'm giving it to God." Live more that way. Everything you do, do for Him, and you will find that it comes back to you a thousandfold.

Yogananda's main message was this kind of love—the love for your own divine potential, first of all, and with that love, the love for other people. In your service, never step beyond that love in the sense that you work with tension, thinking, "I've *got* to do this," and "I *must* do that." Then you get all uptight about it, and that's not service to God. The greatest service you can give God is the simple expression of divine love.

I remember once years ago, when one of the ministers was in charge of the project of building the towers at the

Encinitas Retreat. There was an opening date which was announced in the newspapers, but as often happens, the project was delayed until it looked as if it couldn't possibly get done on time. They were working all night to try to get it ready, and just at the last moment, the person in charge didn't show up. Later when Yogananda saw him, he said, "Where were you?" The man answered, "Sir, I was meditating." Yogananda replied, "Oh, never mind, that's all right." To him, even at a time of great crisis, putting God first was the only thing that really mattered. I don't mean that he approved of being irresponsible, but if it was for God, then he saw that as the highest responsibility.

This is directly opposite to what we usually think, when we say, "I'll get this done, then I'll do that duty, then maybe I'll have a little time for God." You don't get that time. God first. God all the time. Then you will find that everything somehow flows in an amazing way. Without any real effort, you know the answers. You don't have to work nearly so hard for them because, in that attunement that Infinite Consciousness is expressing through you.

All these different currents that make you what you are today will be effortlessly transformed into higher currents. Now it seems so difficult, but it's not at all. The difficulty is just having enough faith to try it. Once you've tried it, you'll see that it gets simpler and simpler. It takes courage, faith, and devotion, yet finally it's nothing, because that's who you are. Then you will know that your own nature is that divine love. This was Yogananda's message—one that he taught, but more importantly, one that he lived every moment of his life.

Chapter Six

Ananda Village—How It Was Started, and Why

"This kind of spirit is something so dynamic and beautiful that it cannot but become a force to be reckoned with in the future because it's a solution to so many of society's problems."

I'd like to address a subject that I haven't ever spoken about at length before—the topic of communities, and the story of my involvement with them. I was born in Rumania, and perhaps it's because I lived in a kind of community in Teleajen that I became interested in this way of life. We were mostly foreigners living near each other, and were a separate group within the larger country.

I also think it's quite possible that many of us at Ananda were living in a community in the astral world, because it seemed like such a natural way of life to many of us. Master said that often the things people create in this world are done to recapture subconscious memories of a perfection that they'd known in the astral world. This seems entirely possible, because so many of us have an instinctive attunement for communities.

So from childhood I had this idea which began to focalize when I was about fifteen. I started thinking how wonderful it would be if a few people who believed in the same things could live apart from the whole society.

I saw two main purposes for this. The first was to help the individuals involved by being able to mix with people who were on their own wavelength; and the second was to benefit society at large by having people concentrate on and develop certain concepts. Once these ideals were developed by a small group, they could then spread out across society generally without losing their focus.

My thinking grew over the years, so that by the time I reached college, it was more clearly defined. Yet really these thoughts had been in my mind latently for a long time before that. In my college years, I began to think about how often the real steps forward in civilization come from a few people with a shared vision who related to one another in a personal way. A good example is the Renaissance in Florence, Italy, where many of the artists knew each other and fed from each other's inspiration. On the basis of their inspiration, the great art of the Renaissance flourished.

I don't think it would have happened if each of those people had been living in a different country, or if there hadn't been some sort of esprit de corps. It was the sense of an artistic community that got them all thinking in these ways. Each would see how the other painted, or sculpted, and think to himself, "No, it would be better if it were this way." So they borrowed, challenged, and competed with each other, and yet together developed a whole new way of looking at life that became an entire philosophy. Their new approach led them to express themselves creatively without letting dogma dictate what they should do. This produced a great sense of freedom, and paved the way, you might say, for the period of Dwapara Yuga that first began in 1700 A.D.

With the great early scientists—Galileo, Copernicus, and Newton—even though each was living in a different town, and they didn't even live exactly contemporaneously, there was also a feeling of kinship among them. There was a sense of, "We are doing something new." That consciousness fed them all, and began a new scientific movement that I don't think any one person could have done.

The flowering of Shakespearean drama in England was a similar situation. We know Shakespeare because he was the best, but there were many others—Marlowe, Fletcher, and Johnson—who helped to make possible the greatness that was Shakespeare. A lot of their poetry, especially that of Marlowe, was exceptionally good. The Lake Poets in England, Wordsworth and others, knew each other. Through their united energy, they generated a kind of magnetism that drew inspirations that don't often come to individuals. They were writing from within, not just copybook stuff, but it was stimulated by their combined energy drawing inspirations that were very special.

The same thing happened in Germany with the music of Mozart, Bach, and Handel. I remember a little ditty we sang in school in England, "Bach and Handel as you know, died and were buried long ago. Born in the year 1685, still they're very much alive." They were born in the same year, and they either knew each other or knew of each other. Again there was a flowering that I don't think would have happened if there hadn't been that kind of group energy.

Sometimes you find somebody born all alone, and who has to slog the whole thing out by himself, but it usually doesn't produce that kind of real power that you get at these different periods we've spoken about. The same thing is true in religion. If Jesus hadn't had disciples, if they hadn't all felt great inspiration, I don't think we'd have Christianity as we know it. It was the same story with Buddha. It was his dedicated followers who spread his teachings and helped create a world religion.

This pattern occurs over and over throughout history. Great movements come when a few people are fired by a new vision, and feed each other. Mind you, most of the people in society are not particularly musical, or religious, or artistic, but they, too, are inspired by the concentrated energy of the few. I use the image of a pyramid to describe how truth is spread, how a broad base of people gradually is affected by the flowering of a special consciousness in the minds of a few geniuses, or a few people really dedicated to helping these things come about.

During those periods, there were many other people that we don't know about today who were also producing creatively in art or music, and they also had their influence. It was a common thing in those days for people to think more in artistic terms, where today people think rather in business or political terms. What I notice in our culture now is that because it's so vast, so multifarious, it's much more difficult to bring ideas to a focus. You read about the warring city-states in the time of St. Francis, for example, and you imagine them as great cities. But when you go there and see them, you think, "My gosh, that was a city?" The wall that enclosed them was so small that really what they had was a small community. There were no big cities as we would consider them today. There were villages or small towns, but in that smallness there was a focus that we don't have in our society.

So it seemed to me, as I began thinking about these things in the late thirties and early forties that more than ever before, we needed small communities that were focused around ideals, not just on economic necessity. We've had plenty of villages that developed because there happened to be a coal mine, or a port, or some other economic opportunity that made people flock there. None of these were based on any ideals, but grew just because there were jobs available.

It seemed essential to show people a way out of the increasing complexity which I didn't see going toward any sense of clarity. It looked likely to me that the Second World War could easily continue into a Third World War, into perhaps global destruction, because there was too much confusion, too many voices, and too little clarity. I felt that not only for the individual, but also for society at large, a new direction was desperately needed. There needed to be a few people who got together and brought clarity to their own lives because they weren't threatened from all sides by so many different definitions of what life is all about. They could create something that would be based in idealism, not just by accident or economic necessity. So, for the sake of society itself, we needed a few people who could bring some clarity out of this chaos.

Recently a friend of ours said, "I think that Ananda is the most important thing happening on this planet." I didn't say what you might expect one to say from an attitude of humility, "I'm glad you think so." I spoke rather from a sense of certainty, and said, "Yes, I know it is." I believe that a hundred years from now people aren't going to look back and think about Clinton, Whitewater, and all the different wars of this century. I think they're going to look at the people who were seeking solutions. It's not that Ananda specifically is *the* important place. It's rather a spearhead, one of several, of something that's happening today showing people a way to the future—a way of life that is based on essential human realities.

One of the big problems today is that people have gotten away from the villages, from a way of life where they knew their neighbors. When life was on a smaller scale, we knew other people better. We knew their problems, and would help them when it was needed. Now we have people living in their millions and millions in big cities where you don't know anybody. You'd think in a crowd it would be impossible to feel isolated, but the problem everywhere is loneliness—not knowing your neighbor, not knowing anyone deeply. We don't know people we can weep with. Perhaps we talk to them socially at a party, but can we share our problems with them? No. We've created social programs to help with this, and those social programs don't work in the same way.

One of the beautiful things about Ananda is that there's such concern for the needs of others. If somebody needs to go to the hospital, for example, everybody pitches in to help that person, so that his bills are paid, and he doesn't have to worry. Individually we don't have a lot of money, but we have a very strong financial base because three hundred and fifty people are there to help do what they can. If a couple gets married, members willingly come forward to give them money for a honeymoon trip. This kind of group cooperative spirit where people all work together and help each other is very rare in this world. Usually the only people you can look to for help are relatives who want their quid pro quo. If you ask them to do anything for you, they're going to ask something back in return, or if they help, it will be with a sense of obligation, not of joy.

Another thing that you run into in typical communities is that when people leave, they're ignored or forgotten. At

Ananda it's not like that. Years ago, long before we became what we are now, there was a couple who decided to leave Ananda. We didn't have the homes we have today, and they were living in a bus. Two weeks before their stated departure date, the bus burned down. They lost everything—all their clothing, furnishings, utensils for cooking, and money. Except for the clothes they were wearing, they were left with nothing. There was no group meeting to decide, "We've got to help these people," or, "Even if they were about to leave, we've still got to be compassionate." There were no big slogans or statements, but perfectly naturally everybody pitched in and gave them money, clothing, pots and pans—everything they needed so that they could leave happily. Nobody ordered that kind of spirit. It just happened because that's the attitude on which our whole community was founded, and still exists today.

This kind of spirit is something so dynamic and beautiful that it cannot but become a force to be reckoned with in the future because it's a solution to so many of society's problems. Today we're living in isolation, in a sense of competition with our neighbors. We're worried about getting ours and, if necessary, we'll take it from theirs. In contrast here are a group of people at Ananda who live in harmony and peace. At first people think it's impossible, but when they see it happening, they begin to think, "Maybe it *is* possible." And, indeed, it is.

Two or three years ago somebody said to me, "You have some wonderful people living at Ananda." He'd just met a few. I said, "If you met only one or two such people, you might say *they* were wonderful, but when you see many people like that, it begs another conclusion. It's *what they're doing* that's wonderful." People change their consciousness when they realize that it really is possible to live supportively in friendship with others, not competing in a cutthroat way, or always putting others down. From a spiritual standpoint, it's a great help to find that this is possible. We all have our ups and downs, but when you're down, what a joy to find there are people around to help lift you up. They know, too, that if they're down, you'll help them out because of the strong desire to help one another.

This is true in all aspects of our lives, and even with the children in our schools. I loved something that one of our children said after a race he ran with children from a neighboring school. Somebody asked him, "Did you win?" He said, "No, but I won against myself," meaning that he beat his own record. How beautiful for an eight-year-old child to understand this! You find that in Ananda schools there is this same kind of cooperative effort to help each other—not to put each other down, which is so normal with children.

This cooperative spirit permeates our spiritual lives, our work within the community, and with the larger community outside Ananda. People in Nevada County, California where we live, love to work with us because they see that we don't think in terms of getting ours—we think in terms of helping them, too. We don't hesitate to bargain with them to get a good deal when we can, but if that bargaining is prejudicial to the other person, we wouldn't dream of doing it.

The influence of what we're doing is also part of a larger picture, part of the synchronicity that you find happening elsewhere, because nobody is just an island. There are many examples of similar things that seem to happen at the same time in history. For example, the principles of leadership that we use at Ananda, and that I wrote a book about, are being used more and more in businesses. I'd like to think that at least some of this new approach has been caused by what I wrote, although I know that the same ideas are occurring to many others. Big companies like Kellogg, Minolta, and AT&T have bought my book, *The Art of Supportive Leadership,* by the hundreds to give out to their managers. More and more people are thinking in terms of leadership as service, as working together with others, and not as a position of importance over others. I don't know how much influence we've had directly, but we're certainly a part of this wave that more and more people are becoming aware of.

When Ananda bought a bookstore, some of the people who started working there were unsure of their ability to run a bookstore. They said, "But we don't know anything about selling books." I said, "That really doesn't matter. Your customers can tell you what they want, but be their friend. Make them feel that this is a place where they're welcome." In fact, it has flourished because of that attitude. Even if they don't want to buy anything, people come in because they feel that they're greeting friends. This is how the villages used to be, but we've gotten away from that in big city life today.

I remember a store in Lugano, Switzerland where there was a sign in the window reflecting just the opposite attitude. Fortunately they took it down after a time, but the sign said, "The things here are not for touching but for buying. If you're not interested in buying, don't take up our time." We are fortunate that America has a very open mentality. I don't think we could have started the prototype for communities in any other country than America, because in crossing the country as pioneers, Americans had to learn to work together. It's not a new concept. We're just bringing it more clearly to the fore in what we're doing here, but this is the very spirit upon which this country was founded.

So picking up our story, I was thinking about where to start a community, and how to do it, and I even got my friends all enthusiastic about it. I considered starting in Argentina because of its vast, undeveloped territory, and thought maybe we should all move there. I even had this fantasy of the world bombing itself back to the caves, and civilization being preserved by a handful of people who would come back and bring lost knowledge and learning to others. But this is the kind of fantasizing that one gets into, especially as a teenager, when he's trying to create a new thing.

But, nonetheless, I was quite serious about communities, and my friends were all enthusiastic until they discovered how very serious I was. Then they all dropped the idea, and I was left alone. I kept thinking about it, however, and I kept coming back to the thought that what would really help society is small foci of new kinds of thinking and of looking at things. This wouldn't come by being in a big city, but from small groups like in Florence, where this new consciousness would be brought to enough focus to be able to spread with greater clarity and magnetism.

If each one of our members lived in a different city, each one might still be meditative and peaceful. In the office where he worked, perhaps everyone might be getting rattled, and this one person remained peaceful. The conclusion that most people would draw from his example is that he's a special kind of person. If he insisted that he was peaceful because of his way of life, they might say, "Well, he probably eats bran for breakfast" , but they wouldn't take it to themselves. They wouldn't think, "Anybody can do it," but they'd still be convinced that he was special. It's when you see a community of people living together in harmony, especially if you knew some of them beforehand , that you begin to think that this is possible for you, too. You begin to think that you could live in peace.

What other way is there to live? It's so wonderful to be able to live among people who are idealistic, who aren't always putting others down. When you turn on the television, what do you see? In the first five minutes, you see somebody shooting somebody, somebody hitting somebody, or somebody insulting somebody. People think that this is normal, but it isn't. It's not normal when we live abnormally. We are souls, we are children of God, and that's the normal way to live.

We need to have enough power behind that statement so that people seeing it will begin to think, "It is possible to live according to my ideals. Maybe I could. Maybe the world could be better." I'm absolutely certain it could be better, but it's communities like Ananda that will make it happen—not new laws, or new movements to force people to think differently. By being that way ourselves, by living as God's children, and by setting that example, we will make a tremendous impact for good on society.

In my early thinking about communities, I hadn't yet added a spiritual component. I wasn't thinking about the spiritual path—I didn't even know there was such a thing as a spiritual path, but like all of us I suppose, I was on it without knowing it. I couldn't get away from the concept of God, though I didn't know what God was. Then I went through an anguishing period trying to understand what life was all about, and finally came to the realization that I needed God. All the self-effort I had gone through for years to uplift myself had been so petty and ineffective. I'd do a little bit here, and then that would fall apart. I couldn't get myself together. I began to realize I needed God's help, and I needed it desperately because I desperately wanted to change.

Then I came upon a book called *The Short World Bible,* which gave excerpts from the different world religions. When I came upon the excerpts from the Hinduism, I thought, "Finally I've found what I've been looking for." Here was something that talked about an infinite truth. It talked not just of a God in a human form, but of an Infinite Consciousness out of which everything has come. This inspired me to my core. I had wanted to be an astronomer because of the inspiration of vastness, and here was a religion that talked about that. Another thing that moved me deeply was the statement that you have to experience these truths for yourself—it wasn't enough just to believe them. I was so sick of being intellectual. I'd fought my way to find these concepts of truth, but it wasn't giving me happiness. It also said in another excerpt, "If you want to know Me, go to a solitary place and meditate on Me." I thought, "All right. Nothing in this world matters a thing to me. I will go off and meditate."

I wanted to be a writer to help humanity, but I realized that I didn't have anything to help humanity with. How could the blind lead the blind? I didn't want to flood the world with my ignorance, so I gave up the thought of writing. Instead I thought, "Let me at least find peace of mind, and then maybe I can help other people." But I had no idea what to do. I'd sit on a bed cross-legged and cross-eyed, and didn't know what was going on, but the Hindu scriptures had said to meditate, so I tried to meditate.

Then I came upon *Autobiography of a Yogi* by Paramhansa Yogananda, and it changed my life so radically that I took the next bus from New York to California. It was one of those beautiful, divine coincidences, if you want to put it that way, because I had just put my mother on a ship to join my father in Cairo where he'd been transferred. The very day that I put her on the ship, I went up to Fifth Avenue and found *Autobiography of a Yogi*. Then I came to Master, and felt that I didn't want anything more except to serve God in my guru's ashram for the rest of my life.

But as I lived with him, and heard him talk to his disciples and to others, my thought of community began to be reawakened, because I found that this was a fundamental interest of his as well. In the present edition of *Autobiography* in the "Aims and Ideals of Self-Realization Fellowship" the passage referring to World Brotherhood Colonies has been removed, but it was something he talked about all the way up to his passing. He was very keen on it. The reason for the removal was strictly because he hadn't been able to get people to understand it yet. Perhaps of all those people who came to him, I was the only one who shared this interest, as if it was something I was born to do. When I asked one of the leaders of the organization, "When are we going to get these communities going?" Her answer was, "Frankly, I'm not interested."

But *I* was. I thought it through long before meeting him, and I would talk to people to get ideas of how to make a community work. I spoke with a financier from Australia to try to get suggestions as to how to make such a thing financially viable. I visited a kibbutz in Israel, and a community in Dalbhag, India. I studied all sorts of things to try to find out how to do this because

I'd read that many communities had been started, and none of them had succeeded. I found, in fact, in the skein of the weaving of American history that communities were a very important part of America's history.

At the very beginning of this country's history, the early settlers had to live in that way. The Pilgrim Fathers founded many intentional communities in their effort to escape religious persecution and find a way to worship God. Although in time many of these communities became dogmatic—this is a human failing—nonetheless, they had initially come together for a higher purpose, not just to carve out of the wilderness some opportunity to live together, but to uphold their ideals.

A man from South America told me something quite interesting. He said, "Do you know why America has succeeded, and South America has not? Because when people came to America, they came for God. When they came to South America, they came for gold. Ever since then, we've known nothing but chaos, political turmoil, and unrest. In America there's been social order and steady growth." Now people are trying to separate God out of the American mentality. By doing that, they're taking the soul out of it, because that's what made America what it is.

Later in the nineteenth century in America, there were many other communities that were started. Some of them didn't survive; some of them, like the Shakers, succeeded and thrived for over a hundred years. If a business were to continue for a hundred years, you wouldn't call it a failure when it ended. I was in New York a few years ago, and New Yorkers have an ironic sense of humor. It was 1979, and I saw a big sign on the building of some business saying: "Since 1978." But you can't call anything a failure when it's lasted as long as the Shaker communities. I don't think many businesses have lasted anywhere near that length of time.

If communities can last long enough to seed other things, that's really all we should expect. I wouldn't want Ananda to be so frozen and against the thought of change that it would stop being a catalyst for new things to develop. It would be terrible if it just endured in rigor mortis, and became moribund in its absolute change-lessness. One way to endure is refuse to change, but then what's enduring? The true spirit dies, and the form becomes ossified. I've read somewhere that America has the second oldest continuous government in the world. The oldest is England. Our constitution is a wonderful document for it to have endured this long. This has happened because it was written in such a way to allow continuous growth and adaptation.

So when I found that Master himself was behind the idea of communities, it fired my already strong enthusiasm. For years I studied what has made communities work, and what has made them fail. I realized that one absolute necessity would be to have monks or nuns to set the ideal of selfless service. Without this, the human tendency, at least at this stage in our social evolution, is to think of what's in it for me, and to think primarily of "I and mine." But when you see a group of people thinking of giving, and not taking for themselves—and you see them happy—then you begin to think, "Maybe I can live that way, too."

One wonderful thing about Ananda has been that it is an experiment in living. Because we've seen the lives of hundreds of people over the years, we see that certain attitudes work well, and others, though they have their rationale, don't bring about happiness. Invariably those people who think, "I've got to get it together for me first, then I can think about other people," never get it together. Those people who think, "I'm living for God, and that comes first," find that somehow everything works well.

There's no reason why it works, but it does work. "Seek ye first the kingdom of God," Jesus said. Seek that kingdom first, and all these things shall be added unto you. Again and again in the history of Ananda, we've seen that for those who gave, everything worked. For those who took, nothing worked.

Master was all for communities, or "World Brotherhood Colonies," as he called them, but it wasn't just because I was a faithful disciple saying, "Yes, Master," that it worked. It was also something that deeply resonated with me. Perhaps if it hadn't, I wouldn't have understood it enough to do anything. I remember at that Beverly Hills garden party that I've mentioned in *The Path,* when he said with incredible power, "Go North, South, East, and West to start colonies." It was the most powerful talk I'd ever heard in my life, and I deeply vowed that I would do everything I could to make that idea a reality.

As I look back over my life with Master, it's become clear to me over time that I have such a loyal nature that I could never have left Self-Realization Fellowship. Once I've given myself to something, some principle, some person, some cause, then that's it forever. I have a very doubting nature, mostly I've doubted myself, but doubt is partly what makes me a decent teacher. If there's any question or doubt that anybody can have, I've probably had it already. I can understand the dilemma from the inside and can sympathize with it.

But this recognition of the need for communities was fundamental to me. I realized this was what society needed, and that this was what I was to do with my life.

I also realized in looking back that Master was training me to work outside Self-Realization Fellowship. He wouldn't say it then because I wasn't ready to think in those terms. To me, my dedication to him was dedication to the work he founded. Dedication to the work he founded absolutely meant being there and nowhere else.

I remember things he used to say that were steering me in the direction of working independently outside of Self-Realization Fellowship. Once I was present when he was talking to Herbert Freed, who was a minister at the church in Phoenix, Arizona. He was giving him some advice on how to run the church, then he looked at us and said, "You have a great work to do." Without my glasses, I couldn't see whom he was looking at, but assumed it was Herbert. I turned to Herbert, wishing him well with this great work, but Master said quietly but very strongly, "It's you I'm talking to, Walter."* After that many times he used to say to me, "You have a great work to do, and you must . . . "; then he'd give me some specific instructions. It wasn't flattery—he was getting me to take a sense of responsibility. I didn't know what he meant, but I knew it was a public work. I knew that he wanted me to go out to other countries. He said he might send me to Germany and other European countries, and perhaps India, but it was always in the line of public work.

I didn't particularly want to be a public speaker. I knew that I had the germ of ability for it, but it didn't mean anything to me. My feeling was rather, "What an easy way to slip into delusion." I remember once Master was talking to a small group of monks about different ministers who'd been doing public teaching, and how it had gone to their heads. I said, "Sir, that's why I don't

*Yogananda used to call J. Donald Walters, "Walter."

want to be a minister." He looked down, and with a very firm expression, said, "You will *never* fall due to ego." I thought, "Thank God for that," but even so I just didn't really feel in tune with it. Once I said that I didn't want to teach, and he said, "You'd better learn to like it—that's what you have to do."

He also put me in charge of the monks in Self-Realization Fellowship. I was unwell at a certain time, and just as I had tried to get him to agree not to make me a minister, I said to him, "Maybe if I weren't in charge of the monks, I'd get better." All he said was, "I'm thinking about it." There was no word of, "You've got to do it. That's your job." He never talked in terms of me being on the Board of Directors, or of being in charge of any specific part of his work. Nor did he ever put me in charge of a particular church. Rather, every Sunday I talked at a different one—Hollywood, Long Beach, San Diego. In other ways, which I don't need to go into in depth, I see in retrospect that he was planning for me to be doing a work outside.

Now I can see that I could never have started a community if I had been in Self-Realization Fellowship, because there's a strict program that everybody there has to follow. I would have had to be a part of that. He told me that my work was lecturing, writing, and editing. He said, "You will make a good editor someday." With regard to writing, I said to him, "But haven't all the books been written that could possibly be done?" meaning that the mission was his writings. He looked a little shocked and said, "Don't say that. *Much* more is needed."

I had to have the freedom to think things through on my own because I was interested in a different aspect of his work. I was always thinking, "How can this mission reach people who don't know anything about it? How can these teachings be explained to people to help them understand it's what they need?" So it was that after I was put out of Self-Realization Fellowship, the thought came to me, "I will serve my guru by manifesting his idea of World Brotherhood Colonies."

But while my mind was satisfied with this direction, my heart wasn't. I wanted to go into seclusion and just drop out because I was suffering very deeply at that time. So though my wish was to withdraw, somehow Divine Mother pushed me into positions where I had to be involved. I first wanted to help others get land and start a community near Auburn, California. I thought, "That's fine. I'm living fifty miles from there. I can go down every now and then, give a little sage advice, and then withdraw into my seclusion." But God didn't let me do that. I had to be right there, and now I see why—things wouldn't have happened if I'd merely given encouragement to others to do it on their own. So bit by bit, through trial and error, through a lot of storms and hardships, Ananda has evolved into a place where people come from all over the world to find out how we do it. But right now most people aren't yet at a point where they can do it on their own.

My whole idea has been to create a model that other people could take and build on their own. I don't even think of Ananda necessarily as a permanent thing. It may be that everybody may go out from there and start other communities, but what I've seen is that it hasn't happened yet. Those who have tried to go out and start other communities haven't yet succeeded. It's no easy thing. People don't understand that you have to know how to work with people before you can create a community. It's not about solar power or some economic theory—it's about understanding people.

There are two principles that have been at the basis of what we've done. One is that people are more important than things, and the other is that where there is adherence to truth, there is victory. Those two things have held us through thick and thin. Many times a decision was made that looked disastrous for the community, but was right for the individuals involved. We've taken the choice for the individuals, and it has worked out well for the whole.

We've tried to make Ananda's growth come as much as possible from the grassroots level, while still guiding it towards the highest potential. Now Ananda is poised on the brink of reaching many people. More and more people are beginning to think, "This is for me. This is the way I want to live." Those who come here and live will find that your lives will be changed, and you'll also help change many hundreds of others.

One of the problems that we faced in the beginning was that the people who came didn't know me, and didn't even know Master. They liked the idea of living close to nature, but there were many different ideas as to what this fledging community ought to be. I didn't want to dictate and say, "You've got to do it this way." I always tried to bring the right direction out of them, so I had to exercise patience. Yet I couldn't allow it to become too diffuse—it had to go in one direction. The hardest test we faced in the beginning was the need for self-definition. It was something that I didn't want to impose on anybody, but had to draw out of them.

This took a little while, but bit by bit people began to see, "Yes, this is what we want. We do want to follow Yogananda's path. We do want to live in spiritual harmony. Spiritual dedication has to be paramount. Everything else will work if it is, and nothing will work if it isn't."

We always had groups of people who saw things differently. But we found that gradually as the vibration of dedication to Yogananda and his principles grew stronger, people who weren't in harmony with that left of their own accord.

Ananda needs to be like water flowing from a mountain if it is to serve as an example for others. If the vision starts from a high peak, then it has the momentum to reach out far into the plains. If, on the other hand, we start at sea level, it would just create a surrounding puddle. We need to come from the heights with the prototype. Later on when other people come, they can take the germ of this idea and do with it what they like. It's bound to have many repercussions, many kinds of influences and ramifications, but at this time we still need that kind of clarity that helps establish a new vision. The rest can happen in its own time.

There was one time when we felt the need for this greater spiritual clarification and dedication, but we weren't sure quite how to make it happen. Fortunately Divine Mother made it happen for us. She sent a forest fire that destroyed twenty-one of our twenty-two homes, and destroyed four hundred and fifty of our seven hundred acres. Those who didn't have dedication left—there was no problem. But those who did have it didn't take the fire as the tragedy that you'd normally assume. To them it was an opportunity. There's a lovely picture of one of our members, Asha, the day after the fire striding through those smoking logs to clear the land so that we could build again. We didn't have insurance or any savings. To everyone else, it seemed certain that we would fail, but not to us.

Right after the fire, our neighbors made a discovery and phoned us, all excited about it. They found that the fire had been caused by a faulty spark arrester on a County vehicle. Our neighbors enthusiastically sued the County, got their money back, and were able to rebuild even without insurance. I wrote to the County Supervisors, and said, "I know that you're worried that we're going to sue you because we were the major loser in this fire. I want you to know that we will not sue. We came here to give, not to take our bad luck out on others." I think it took them a few years of waiting for the other shoe to drop, but it never did. Making money by suing others is to me an unrighteous thing to do. I would rather fail and adhere to our principle, "Where there is adherence to truth, there alone is victory." Ten years later our neighbors were still weeping over what they'd lost, and we flowered.

We found that every major test—and Ananda has had its share—has been the precursor to a flowering period such as we'd never been able to have without tests and difficulties. Now we can look back on the challenges and say that they were wonderful—they helped make us stronger and more clear in what we're trying to do. Ananda isn't a fixed thing or a crystallized form, but an ever-growing movement within the vision of Master, our line of gurus, and of their ray of consciousness. I couldn't have done it without their help. It was because I was trying to work in attunement with them that many miracles have happened along the way. God had only to withhold one important miracle for Ananda not to exist anymore. It has taken divine help, and lots of it, but it's also taken our willingness and dedication.

I would like to say to all those who think about living in a spiritual community that for your spiritual growth and the growth of the world, this is a marvelous thing to do. Quite honestly, I don't think a day goes by that I don't think, "What a wonderful way to live!" Yes, there are tests. Yes, there are difficulties. So what's new about that? Life is like that, but what a great thing to have so many real friends who would give their lives for you. The more we grow in that spirit, the better example we will be to others.

Another problem you find in communities is what Krishna talked about in the *Bhagavad Gita* when he said to his disciple, Arjuna, "You who have overcome the carping spirit, to you I reveal these truths." There always arises one of the problems of human nature—the carping spirit, the thought that things are okay, but they could be better if they were another way. People are always trying to find some fault with the way things are being done.

We used to have a lot of this when we were starting Ananda. In fact, in the beginning it seemed that I had only to open my mouth for half the community to jump down it. In the early days, people had the thought, "We're here for God. We just want to meditate. We want to live a spiritual life. Why do we have to think about money? God will take care of us." God does take care of you, if you make the effort, but if you're going to sit back and let Him do it all, He's not going to do anything for you. He helps those who help themselves. So I said, "I understand. It's taken me years to come to this point of realizing the need for being practical. I don't expect you to have leapt to that conclusion immediately, so I will go out and work for a year to pay the mortgage. But after that, on May 31, 1970, I will come back here, and by then I will expect you to have reached this understanding."

I began giving yoga and meditation classes in a different city every night to try to raise the money that was needed each month. This was difficult because there was no income beyond what I brought in through teaching. All I had was my own efforts, my belief in the vision of communities, and, of course, the most important thing—Master. But all that was behind the scenes. I remember one evening I returned to Ananda and had a satsang with everyone there. I gave a talk about how we've got to start businesses that will support Ananda, and they became furious. They thought I was being a materialist, and they were being spiritual. Their spirituality amounted to a little bit of meditation, and then going down to the Yuba River to swim. I think the most difficult thing for me to accept was they saw my willingness to work for them as the justification of their philosophy that God would take care of them.

Shortly after that I got a letter from the trustees saying we had to pay our back payments, or they would foreclose in two weeks. I argued that since they hadn't yet honored their agreement of putting in new roads, we shouldn't have to pay. Their letter said, "We understand how you would feel this way, but the law doesn't force us to honor a verbal agreement. We're going to foreclose in two weeks if you can't pay in full." This meant coming up with a great deal of money we didn't have. The only time that I can remember being nervous was that night. We had a little center in Sacramento, California, and the minister there said, "Come to the center and have some tea. You'll feel better." I said, "I don't care how I *feel* about this thing. I want to know what to *do* about it."

Even though it was quite late, when I got home I began calling people on the phone to see if they could help us out in this. I spent my free time making recordings to sell and perhaps generate a little bit of money.

With God's grace, the day before the payment was due, I was able to send the check in and save the day.

I moved up to Ananda on May 31, as I had said. Thankfully by this time, others had also decided that they would help generate the money. One of the founding members, Jyotish, started an incense and oils business, and others started things to help out financially. One month later, on July 4, our temple burned to the ground. It was quite an interesting thing, because a few months later a friend and I were talking about the tests and difficulties that people go through. With all sincerity, I said, "You know, it's strange, but my life doesn't seem to have any tests." She said, "Oh my God," and started listing all the things that she'd experienced with me in the one year of Ananda. I said, "Oh yes, I guess that's so."

But I think one of the things that has helped us is that I've never accepted problem consciousness. I've always been determined to find solution consciousness and to embrace it. So I didn't think of these tests as great setbacks. They happened. Let it be. My response has always been, "What do we do about it?" So in the early years, people would pose problems or have criticisms, and my answer was, "Give me a solution. Otherwise, I don't want to hear about it."

One basic understanding I've had which has helped make Ananda work has been the willingness to work with people who wanted to help build, and not devote a lot of energy to people who are merely negative. I believe that if you work with negative people with a great deal of patience and energy, you may bring them to zero, but then what have you got? It's far better to concentrate on those people who really want to work together. Just as we said earlier, it's through the focused energy and magnetism of a few that real changes are made.

We need to help Ananda to grow always in the direction of principles rather than of banners and slogans. We need the principles of love, tolerance, kindness, truth, self-control, and concern for the welfare of others. Our community is not just the people living there—our community is our neighbors. Beyond that, Ananda is a community of truth-seekers living throughout the world, seeking a better way of life based on their ideals.

Somebody recently said to me, "It was easy for you to start a community, but it's very difficult now." No, it was not particularly easy, but it was a joy. Would I do it again? Yes, I would. Knowing all the problems we've had to face? Yes, I would. Master said, "God is our stocks and bonds." God is our strength. What it has taken to build Ananda will continue, because now many others understand the principles of how to do it. The spirit that Master instilled in me, and through me to all of you, will be instrumental in creating a new and better world. If we can serve God, have the joy of living for Him, and sharing Him with others, what great fulfillment can there be?

Chapter Seven

How to Be a True Disciple

"More than just being a student or being willing to take discipline, try deeply to tune in to the guru as the spoken voice of silent God, as the manifested ray of the effulgent light of the Infinite. Through that attunement, you will find more and more that you absorb within yourself that Infinite Light, and you become divine."

There are two words that come to mind when we think of discipleship—the first is "student." What is implied by this word? Obviously, "study" which means learning, memorizing, trying to understand with the intellect, and putting things together like a jigsaw puzzle until it finally makes sense.

Most people who come to a teacher—whether he be an artist, a musician, a composer, or indeed, a spiritual teacher—come in the capacity of student. When Master talked to students and to the general public, he went to great length to explain spiritual principles—what to do in order to advance spiritually, why these practices are necessary, and even why you need to take up the spiritual path. In other words, he approached it from the outside in.

In the same way, people who go to art school can learn all the different techniques that artists have used, ways of mixing color, the principle of symmetry, and the kinds of artistic theories that have been held over the centuries. Hundreds, probably many thousands, of people graduate from art school every year, and many become competent advertising or display artists. By no means all do so, but generally speaking anybody with a certain level of talent and intelligence will reach a competent level of skill.

But great artists are few. Not many people who graduate from art school go on to become exceptional artists. Some who are truly great may even remain unknown, but still they are prominent in the eyes of truth. One of the ironies of the whole system of education is, if you read the lives of great geniuses, you find that many of them have done badly in school, or haven't even gone to school. Sri Yukteswar was quite slow in his studies, because he wasn't very interested. Master was so far from interested that he spent most of his time in his guru's ashram, and passed his exams by the skin of a few blessings, you might say. Yet he absorbed something else of far greater importance.

The second meaning of the word disciple is someone who takes it up as a serious discipline. He is willing to inwardly absorb the subject, and to make something of himself in the process. He is willing to take on the mantle of art, or of yoga, or of whatever he's been studying, and to approach it more from the inside out. When Master talked to his disciples, those who lived in the ashrams and who had already committed their lives to him, he didn't talk nearly so much on a level of philosophy. In fact, often he would go on for hours with guests, but he wouldn't talk at all to the disciples. If he did talk, it was just a little hint, a phrase—it was something to meditate on for many years before you really understood it.

I find that in my years with Master (I came to him in 1948, so it's going on 50 years), I've been not only his student, but more than that—I've been his disciple. I've spent all these years meditating on the things that he did and said, and have tried to understand them by getting behind his actions and words into the spirit that motivated them. In other words, I've tried to understand him from within. This is discipleship, and it means taking discipline.

When I came to him, he asked two things of me. First, he said, "I give you my unconditional love," and he asked that of me. Then he also asked me to give him my unconditional obedience. This was something I wasn't sure about, even though I was desperate to be accepted. In my mind I was saying, "You just *have* to accept me," but still I wanted to be honest. So I said, "But suppose, Sir, I should ever think you wrong?" He said, "What I tell you to do won't be my desire or opinion. I will say it because God tells me to say it." How could I reply to that? I gave him my unconditional obedience on the basis that I would certainly follow him as the voice of God.

This is what it is to follow the guru, and to have the kind of obedience that doesn't say, "Well, my guru said this, but St. Francis or Ramana Maharshi said something else." It means having that level of intuition that says, "I know this is for me." I have to say that, although I've had a doubting nature, one doubt I've never had for a split second is, "Is Master my guru? Is he mine or not?" I knew from the moment I met him that he was mine. If anybody tried to persuade me that another one was greater, it didn't matter—mine could be second best, but he was mine.

This attitude of openness on the disciple's part makes it possible to have that level of intuition to know what it is you're receiving. This intuition doesn't come by will power or by anything except grace. But again, this grace isn't given to certain people because of something in their personality, or because they've somehow phrased their prayers in just the right way. Nor does it come because they've been diplomatic enough in their self-presentation to God that He says, "Okay, you I'll listen to." No, He watches the heart. When He knows that your longing for Him is deep enough, then He will give you the grace of faith. Pray for this grace that enables you to know your own way, to know what is yours. You can't will yourself into this attitude, but you can pray for it and open yourself to it.

We need to understand that God comes in many different ways. St. Simeon the New Theologian, a great Christian saint of the Tenth Century, made an important point in this regard. Even though he lived a thousand years ago, he was called "the New Theologian" in his time, and the name has stuck. Anyway, he made a very strong point of saying that the teachings of the Bible are to be understood from those who are living it in their own day and age. He scolded people who kept comparing the spiritual teachings of his time with the teachings of people several centuries ago.

You find that many people who come onto the path say, "Yes, one saint might have said this, but St. Francis, or Jesus, or Buddha said that." They make comparisons whereas, in fact, truth is one. You can't change truth—all you can do is change its presentation. Once I asked Master, "Is this a new religion you've brought?" He said, "It is a new expression." Truth remains the same. You can't have one God with one truth here, and another one with a different truth on a mountain top over there. No, it's one truth, and one God.

In your study of the history of religion, it's of primary importance to understand that fact. The scholars will tell you Shankaracharya was against Buddha, and Buddha was against the Vedas, and on and on. This is just a bunch of mischief—it's not the truth. Study the saints primarily from the point of view that there is one truth that they're expressing. Here is a guideline I always use in considering a teaching: Is it in keeping with the tradition of the ancients? Those traditions will never change. Whether we're flying jet engines or riding camels, truth remains unchanged.

But there are saints who at various times have explained things in different ways in order to help people understand them better. When I was new on the path I used to think that the way things were phrased in scripture was inherently spiritual. Remember that at one time scripture was composed by living people in flesh and blood with all the problems common to mankind. It's the ancient phraseology and metaphors that make you think, "Wow, this is something great." Instead of using the language of today that we're accustomed to, scripture is written in an archaic way that has an aura of dignity about it. You don't expect Jesus to use words like "shucks," but he used his equivalent. It's not that I ever heard Master use that word, but it came to mind.

Master spoke modern English, and it could be pretty salty at times, depending on the needs of the audience. The way he expressed the teachings was in tune with contemporary culture—Madison Avenue, Hollywood, cars, and airplanes. It doesn't seem to have the aura of scripture, but someday it will. We must understand that the way God has expressed himself today is the way He's *always* expressed himself, but it changes outwardly according to the needs of the times. If St. Francis lived it differently, that was because his times were different. The needs of today, the needs of a particular country, and the needs of a particular individual asking a question— all these things need to be taken into account when expressing the teachings. So don't think, "How does what these people say jibe with what was said a long time ago?" It will not change; it cannot change. It is only given an emphasis that is more meaningful today.

There was a time in the Christian religion when all those who really wanted God went out into the desert. Does that mean we should all go out into the desert to find God? Maybe, but maybe not. In fact, Yogananda didn't guide us toward that particular way of life, though he might have emphasized it for a specific individual. Don't think that because the Desert Fathers totally withdrew from civilization and Master didn't stress it that, therefore, one way is holier or better than the other. It's only different because the needs then were different from the needs now. In those days it was descending Kali Yuga, when peoples' consciousness was moving increasingly toward spiritual darkness. The only way to rescue anything from that trend was to go off and just be with God.

Now we're in an upswing of civilization, ascending Dwapara Yuga, where people can understand that it's possible to bring these truths into our daily lives. This is why Lahiri Mahasaya lived the life of a householder. Once when somebody criticized Trailanga Swami, a great Indian saint and contemporary of Lahiri, for giving such reverence and honor to him, he said, "Lahiri Mahasaya has attained that which I have renounced even my loincloth to find." Lahiri Mahasaya was a master of the highest stature. He was much greater than Trailanga Swami who, though a great saint himself, wasn't yet fully liberated at that time. The point is to look to the saints of this day. Don't look nostalgically to the past, but draw from those saints of today who are giving you what you need now.

There are some saints that I met in India who, though I know them to be great souls, were just not for me. They didn't resonate with my consciousness or my spiritual needs. God sends many different saints into the world so that those with one kind of temperament will be satisfied, and those with a different nature will find their way as well. As Ramakrishna put it, "Everybody likes sweetness, but some like it in the form of chocolate, some in the form of honey, and some in the form of sweetmeats." Ramakrishna, for example, was a great saint, but he's not my way. Yogananda *is* my way, and this is the point of understanding we need to begin with.

If we're going to pray for that faith to know our own, we must understand that it isn't a matter of personality. A certain ray comes into the world, and expresses itself through different masters according to the needs of the times, the particular country, and the group of disciples. Each divine ray is like a rainbow. Though it has seven colors, it's all one light. The spectrum in the spiritual plane has many, many gradations, and not one of them is better or worse than another.

The important thing is not to think in terms of personality, because a master, or even a great saint, will have many different types of disciples. It's on a deeper level than intellect. You just know without questioning which is your way. Once you really know that, then don't look left or right. People say, "You need to find a guru," but God makes that decision, not us. What you have to recognize is, "This is what God wants for me. This is my way." Once you have that, then you move from the ranks of student and become a real disciple.

Students are many. They begin as curiosity seekers who think, "It might be a good thing to do something besides go to cocktail parties. I'll set aside one day a week to go to a lecture and see how I like it." Then they think, "This is pretty hot stuff. Let's see what other people talk about." So they go to many lectures, read different books, study one self-help method after another, and it all sounds very exciting. Often they feel elated because they've finally gotten out of one problem, but then they wake up the next day or the next week to find that they've got another. They've only moved from one room in the house of ego to another. People go around from one new method to another, but they stay in that same house.

The only reason they feel better is that they've returned to the state they had before they were aware of the problem. It's just like when you pinch the flesh on your hand—it hurts, but when you finally let go, it feels so good. Perhaps you were obsessed with some problem you had with your parents when you were young, and finally you come to terms with them and feel better. You can accept them and realize they, too, had their problems. In fact, you realize that you're not really all that different from them anyway. You feel much better about the situation, but are you therefore liberated? Far from it! You now begin looking at other problems—perhaps your professors, or your neighbors, or your boss didn't treat you right. You continue on and on in this way until finally you've come around the house, and in the next incarnation it's your parents again!

The way out of this, of course, is to get out of the ego. Once you've come out of the house, *then* you're liberated.

That alone is the state of lasting joy and peace. People who wander a great deal, going to lecture after lecture and path after path, never find this. They think, "This guy says he's great, so he must be great. This guy says he's greater, so he must be greater. And this guy was written up in the *Wall Street Journal,* so he must be fantastic." It's understandable to think this way at first, and I'm not criticizing it. We all have to go through these different phases, just as you have to go through different grades in school. One of the grades of spiritual advancement is looking around and comparing various ways—I even recommend it to people. If you don't feel certain about your path, then one way to know is to compare a bit. But once you begin to feel that you've found your way, then don't look anymore, because you'll just go in circles. You need to say, "This way is mine," and then you become a student on a different level. You realize that though many different paths may be true, on the level of human understanding, they just present a conflict. One saint says, "Stay in seclusion," while another says, "Work in the world." A third saint says, "Study the scriptures," and the next says, "Don't study anything but just chant." You find a lot of contradictions in spiritual teaching, and on a mental level it's confusing. If you read all sorts of books and try to draw your truth from them, you won't have any truth to draw—you'll just be confused.

It's far better to go deeply into one path, one teacher, and one teaching. Master said, "If you do even a hundredth of what I tell you, you'll find God." Great masters give us a great variety of disciplines partly to show us how urgently we need to seek God, and partly to satisfy the varying needs of different disciples. Some will be helped by guidance and training in one direction, and some by another.

Once you know your own way, then become a deep student, not of abstract or intellectual truth, but of the teaching of that particular guru. Discipleship is more than absorbing ideas. It's tuning in to the ray of consciousness that God has sent you. There's a very good story to illustrate this. St. Augustine, who had written some of the greatest theology in the history of Christendom, was out one day walking on the beach. He saw a little child about three years old repeatedly going down to the sea to fill a bucket with water, and then coming up onto the sand and emptying it. This was an unusual enough practice that St. Augustine stood there and watched him for some time. Finally he said to the child, "Don't you realize you can never empty the sea with that little bucket?" The boy looked up at him, and with amazing wisdom said, "Isn't it just as strange for you to think that you can empty the sea of wisdom with your little mind?" Then he vanished. St. Augustine knew that it was a divine manifestation sent to teach him this lesson.

You can never understand truth with your brain, no matter how intelligent you are. You could have the intelligence of a hundred Einsteins put together, and you'd still never understand it. All the amazing things that individuals have been able to accomplish, you, too, could do if you applied yourself in the same way. It might take you many incarnations, just as it took them, to get to that level of genius, but the potential is there within you. We don't do it with our brain—we receive it. The greatest acts of genius have always been received from that Infinite Ocean—nobody creates it. Even after a lot of thinking, the greatest insights of genius are received in a flash. You suddenly understand, and you didn't need a lot of thinking to reach them. Mainly what the thinking does is to push aside the confusion so that you are open to receive.

But any ray of the Divine that is expressed by a master will still be a limited thing because the Divine is infinite, and *beyond* infinite. Even though a master is one with the Infinite, one with God, while he's in a human body he can only express a certain aspect of that consciousness to his students. But remember that in attuning to that ray, it's like entering the tip of an inverted pyramid. You enter at the point which is at the bottom, and then as you come up, the pyramid increasingly spreads out until you become one with all there is. That ray of the Divine brought by a master will not limit you—it was meant to give you entry to the Infinite. You can't enter a building through the wall. You have to find the door that leads inside and go through it. Then you have access to the whole building.

Don't think, "Oh, but I haven't learned about the ancient Egyptian mysteries. I haven't studied the Chaldeans." These are all different things that people who go by theory like to get into. Realize that none of these things are going to take you into the building or give you real wisdom. All this learning will do is fill your brain with a lot of useless information. I'm reminded of an episode from one of the Sherlock Holmes stories. Watson, his trusty helper, mentioned to him some very simple fact that everybody knows, like the Earth going around the Sun, or Mars having two satellites. Watson was surprised that Holmes, with all his knowledge as a detective, didn't know this fact. Holmes's reply was, "Now that I know it, I'm going to try to forget it immediately, because this knowledge is useless to me in my profession as a detective."

So it is that we need to simplify our knowledge. We confuse our minds by overburdening them with useless furniture, like stuffing an attic with so much clutter that it's impossible to move around in. We need to simplify our lives, our brains, and our intellects as well. Once you understand this, then you begin to really zero in on what *your* teacher taught. Then you're ready for a guru, but not until then. When you've got that kind of consciousness, then the Divine takes an interest in you. When I came to Master, I had no idea that Divine Mother was interested enough in my case to tell him to see me even though he wasn't seeing anybody because his appointments were filled for two months.

God takes an interest when you take an interest—it's as simple as that. It isn't that He says, "Here's somebody who's really smart. I'm going to choose him." No. If you long for that help, then God says, "All right, I'll help you." He wants to help you, but He can't help you if your eyes are on the ground. How then are you going to see the light of His star? It has to come from your openness, your longing for God, your willingness to follow Him, and your desperation to find the truth without wasting any more time. When you reach that point, then you're really ready to be a disciple of a guru, and that is when the guru is going to become interested. Mind you, God sends the guru, but he won't lead you until you have that depth of real commitment. When you have it, the guru will take charge of your life.

You need to go still deeper for the guru to say, "I'm going to hang on to this person until he finds freedom." That's an even deeper kind of commitment, so it all depends on your commitment, not his. But once that ray enters your consciousness, something else happens. There was a printer at Mt. Washington who was a worldly man and not at all interested in spiritual truths. He was hired to print the books, and he used to spend a fair amount of time joking about these yogis with their meditation and their idea of a guru. It was all nonsense to him, but one of the monks there took it upon himself to befriend him and explain the teachings to him. He began to think, "This sounds pretty good," and he began to notice that the people around him were really kind and loving.

Finally Master saw that he was starting to open up, so he called him upstairs for an interview. I don't think Master said anything much. It was probably just the usual kind of superficial things that you ask people when you don't know what to say: Was he married? Did he have children? He may have said more, but here's what really happened. At a certain point Master held this man, Orville, by the sides of the head and looked deeply into his eyes for a long time. When Orville came out, he was just dizzy and didn't know what had happened. But the next time I saw him, he was a devotee. That contact had been made, and it was deep and permanent.

Now this is what we need to pray for—to have that kind of attunement with the ray God has sent us. You see, discipleship goes beyond our word "discipline," which has certain connotations that aren't quite adequate. Discipline brings to mind taking it on the chin, and being willing to correct yourself again and again until you finally get it right. All this is certainly a part of discipleship, but there's another thing that comes in. In India they have two words for disciple: *sishya*, which means "student," and *chela,* which is related to the word for "child." You become a child of the guru—his son or daughter. When that kind of bond is formed, no matter how many lives you stray or struggle, he's still with you.

He will always watch over you and see that you get out of delusion.

This comes not from his choice, nor from anybody else's choice, but your own. You need to pray for it! It's not an intellectual decision, but one that comes from the soul. Once you've said in your heart, "I belong to you, and you belong to me. Nothing else matters but that I am yours." Then no matter what anybody says, you know. The important thing is that you have total attunement and commitment to that ray.

When Master was with his disciples, he often didn't talk very much. Of course, he expressed spiritual truths—he would have to. I was with him for the last three and a half years of his life, which isn't very long, but it's more than the disciples got to spend with Jesus. During that time I found that what he talked of primarily was attunement. He said, "Be in tune. Get in tune. Hang on to that feeling of attunement, and everything will go right." He told us that even if we have many tests and trials in life, our attunement would get us through. In fact, he promised us that there *would* be tests and persecution, because that's a part of the spiritual path. It's how we grow, but if you are in tune, nothing else really matters.

You can understand a subject like painting, for example, from the outside, but that won't make you a great painter. Very few people understand the germ of what it takes to be a painter. Somebody who was with Leonardo da Vinci and studied *him*—not as a man, but his consciousness—in time would be able to paint as well as Leonardo. In fact, da Vinci gave the job of finishing some of his works to those few of his students who had real attunement with his way of painting. He didn't need to do it all, because he did it through them. He'd given them the germ of insight that would enable them to finish the painting in the way he would.

Every great teacher, even of a worldly sort—an artist, a mathematician, or a composer—longs to find a few people who will try to understand the one thing that cannot be conveyed in words, or in a book, or even in a set of principles. He can teach eightfold paths, or tenfold paths, or anything you like, but it will all be superficial. The one real key is to get what he has to convey through inner attunement, or to put it more the way it really happens, the disciple has got to *take* it. The guru always has it there, and he wants to give it to all. But you're the one who has to come in and say, "I take this." At that point, you'll often find that the guru becomes quite shy because he wants to be *sure* you want it. He'll run away from you and hide, as it were.

There's a story of Yogananda when he was a boy at school that illustrates this point. He was sitting in class and wrote a note to a boy next to him saying, "I am your guru." The boy looked at him and said, "Bad boy." Later that night the boy had a vision in which God showed him this was the truth. The next day he went looking for Yogananda to throw himself at his feet, but Yogananda hid. Now he had to find him. You'll find there's always this play of hide-and-seek with God. Once you really understand and want Him, then it seems as if He hides from you because He wants you to desire Him more. When you really seek Him with that kind of intensity, then of course He reveals Himself.

Sometimes you'll find that people who are new on the path will have spiritual experiences that others who have been on the path longer don't have. It's because in the beginning God gives them these things to entice them and make them want Him more. There was one woman who came for the first time to a class that Yogananda was giving in Boston. That evening she saw the thousand-petaled lotus and even saw through the walls of the room. It was an incredible thing, but she never came back!

Years ago I heard about a disciple of Master's in Paris who'd had a terrible experience practicing Kriya Yoga. I thought, "I've never heard about anybody else having a bad experience doing Kriya. I'd like to talk with this man and find out what's going on." Finally the opportunity presented itself when I went to Paris on a lecture tour, and I met him. As soon as he saw me, he called me into a room and sat me down to tell me about his terrible experience. He'd had to give up Kriya and just couldn't practice it anymore. Well, of course, I was all ears! He said, "I was sitting there doing Kriya, and all of a sudden I saw this round light with a star in the middle! I felt myself going into the star and losing myself!" We should all have those problems.

But it's no joke. It takes time to prepare the mind to receive, as Master called it in *Autobiography of a Yogi,* "the liberating shock of omnipresence." This man was having a spiritual experience that he wasn't quite pre-pared to receive. It's not easy to understand the process of inner unfoldment—you have to go by gradual stages. It's not a simple matter of the guru saying, "This person's not ready." It takes time to get ready, but you're the one who has to prepare yourself for the experience. Don't think that God's going to dump it on you—He won't. The more you want it, the more He'll seem to withdraw, so that you want it even more. Once a disciple said to Master, "I call to God with so much longing. Why doesn't He come?" Master said, "That's what makes it so sweet when He does come." You have to want it with *all* your heart, and then He will come easily.

Once when Master was at the Dakshineswar Kali temple, he was praying and praying for Divine Mother to appear, but She didn't reveal herself. Finally they were about to close the doors, and he prayed with extra urgency. Then at last She appeared. Master said that God sometimes tests a devotee to see if he or she really wants Him, and then He manifests. This is typical of the path. When you have that kind of longing, He can't resist you. You are as important to Him as Jesus Christ, Buddha, or any of the great saints who have ever lived. It's not your unworthiness that keeps Him from you—it's your lukewarm devotion. When you want Him and Him only, then He will come. He has to come, because it's God's nature to give Himself.

Here's an example of how the inner attunement of a disciple with his guru works. Master told us that when he was studying Patanjali's *Yoga Sutras,* Sri Yukteswar would keep him working on one stanza for weeks at a time. They went for months before they even reached the eighth stanza. Finally Sri Yukteswar closed the book and said, "Now you've got the key. From now on, any scripture you open can be unlocked with that key."

What I've found over the years is that when I want to do something, I don't just think, "What did Master do in this or that situation?" I tune in to his spirit, and when I feel that spirit, then I know what I should do. Often at that time thoughts and memories of things he said or did that corroborate my feeling come to me spontaneously. Then I have to use my will power to think about things he may have said that contradict what I feel. It's important to do this because the mind can very easily fool itself, and I want to know the truth. If having found a contradiction, I can't rationalize it, then I'm not so sure, and I back off.

You'll find, too, that if you tune in to his spirit, you will understand things far better than if you spend years poring over his writings and studying all the things he said. It's a matter of attunement. That attunement is what will take you to the divine shores.

Here we are—trapped in the ego. Even when we affirm, "I'm free," it's still the ego that's affirming its freedom. How can we free ourselves from the ego when it's bound by its own limitations? This is why a guru is necessary. God could do it directly, but He does everything through channels, so He works through the guru. What transforms us is not his words or his teachings, but his consciousness. You must invite his consciousness into your own. We need to understand this on a subtle level, because I'm not talking about personality. The disciples of a great master are very different from one another, and each one has a certain spark, a magnetism, which makes him truly himself. Through tuning into the guru's consciousness, you will be more truly yourself, rather than suddenly becoming another personality.

But only somebody who is not in the ego will be able to take you out of ego consciousness—that is the role of the guru. There are even some gurus who never speak. You might think, "How can he be a teacher?" It's because speaking isn't really essential to teaching. What is essential is the transfer of consciousness. In *Autobiography of a Yogi,* Master tells how Sri Yukteswar touched him on the chest, and suddenly he went into *samadhi.* Someday just by His touch, God through the guru will liberate you from ego consciousness. You'll be taken out of that into an altogether different kind of consciousness, and you'll see things in a completely new way.

More than just being a student or being willing to take discipline, try deeply to tune in to the guru as the spoken voice of silent God, as the manifested ray of the effulgent light of the Infinite. Through that attunement, you will find more and more that you absorb within yourself that Infinite Light, and you become divine.

Somehow you can see which path the disciples of different gurus follow. Once in New Delhi at the end of a lecture, somebody asked me which path I felt he should follow. He said, "There are no ashrams of Yogananda in New Delhi, so where should I go?" I said, "There's an Aurobindo ashram here. Why not try that?" Then rather surprised, he said, "How did you know that I'm a student of Aurobindo's teachings?" I didn't know, but I did know—it was his ray. Though it wasn't what I would normally recommend to people, it seemed right for him.

Another time, many years ago, somebody called me on the phone to take a class in meditation that I was giving. I could tell from the tone of her voice that she was studying Maharishi's Transcendental Meditation. I asked her what path she was following, and sure enough she was doing TM. I don't know how I knew it, but it's an intuition that I had because people show the ray they're drawing from. When you look at the people from Ananda, even though they're all different, there's something that ties them together, particularly those who are serious about it.

So the attitudes of a disciple are humility, openness, receptivity, and willingness. Be willing to do what you're asked to do, rather than thinking of all the reasons why you shouldn't. You'll find that, in doing this, you'll understand more and more clearly who you are on a deep level.

Remember one thing for a certainty—you are not your personality. You are not your body, male or female. You are not all the things you like and dislike. You are not the things you feel with the human personality you're living through. You are that formless soul—that alone is who you are. The body you take on is just the product of all the things you've done and the reactions you've had over many, many lifetimes. These things have molded your face, your personality, and your likes and dislikes. When you say that you do what you like, what makes you so sure that what you like is something you're so free about? You've developed those likes and dislikes through many situations over incarnations, but you are none of those things.

You are an immortal spark of the Infinite, though you may take on particular accoutrements in any one lifetime. You take on those things to help you get out of this narrow self-definition and to discover that you are the Infinite. You are that Divine Consciousness who is in all personalities and who has taken on all the bodies in the universe. That is what you really are, and it is the God-ordained work of the guru to bring his true disciples to this realization.

Chapter Eight

A Cosmic Vision of Unity

"This vision of seeing the unity in all things doesn't come from putting two disparate things together. It's recognizing that underneath each wave, which seems different in size, shape, and movement, there is the one ocean."

I want to talk about one of the great events of this century—the coming of a soul whose special mission was to show the world a vision of divine unity. As it says in the *Bhagavad Gita*, in every age when darkness increases and virtue declines, God sends one of his enlightened children into the world to inspire mankind in the way of truth. This inspiration comes on many levels.

In one way it offers people the example of an ideal human being who addresses the spiritual needs of that particular age. Such an ideal person came in the form of Buddha with his compassion and world renunciation. When we read about his path of moderation, we must understand that this was a moderation of extremity rather than one of lukewarm spirituality. He was a man of absolute dedication to the quest for *nirvana*, divine consciousness and soul freedom.

Jesus came into this world with a different expression of the Divine. Each one of these enlightened beings has a different kind of personality, not just because God is always new in His expression, but also because every human being, every thumbprint, is a unique creation.

Every personality is unique, but a master doesn't *have* a personality so much as he *manifests* a personality.

Yogananda used to say, "I killed Yogananda long ago. No one dwells in this temple now but God." Indeed, looking into his eyes it was very difficult to see a personality, which in most people is distinguished by the things they like and dislike or in terms of their desires and antipathies. When you looked into his eyes, you didn't see anything of that nature. You saw behind them that deep calmness and infinite consciousness of a soul merged with God. It was truly like being in the presence of God, yet at the same time knowing that his form wasn't God. No form could define God, and yet God is manifest in all beings.

It's important to remember what Jesus said when they accused him of blasphemy for saying that he and God, his Father, were one. He replied to their accusations, "Don't the scriptures say, 'You are gods'?" He didn't say, "God says so, and you'd better believe Him, or you'll go to hell." He didn't justify himself in terms of his own uniqueness, but in terms of *our* divine potential. Then he made it clear that the difference is that he was awake in that consciousness, whereas the generality of mankind is still asleep.

When a master comes into this world, he doesn't come as a person. He comes as a messenger—as a window onto the Divine. I'll give you an illustration in this regard. Many years ago I was working in an office which had a window on the ground floor looking out onto a very beautiful garden. Because my desk faced this garden, I would look up throughout the day to feast my gaze on the flowers, the greenery, and the trees to calm my mind and energize my thoughts.

One day there was a big rainstorm, and mud splattered all over the window so that it wasn't pleasant to look through it. All you saw were the splotches of mud. Two or three weeks passed, and I didn't have the time to clean it, until finally I had a free Saturday and went out and washed the window. Then I came back inside, and said, "Oh, what a beautiful window!" I caught myself and laughed, because I realized what made the window beautiful was the fact that I could no longer see it. I could see through the window, and it no longer obstructed the view of the garden.

Another illustration is found in watching the clouds on the western horizon as the sun is going down. They take on magical hues of gold, red, orange, and sometimes even green. Yet a few minutes later after the sun sets, those same clouds become gray, dark, and uninteresting. So it is with every human being—we are all made radiant by the Divine Light within us. Each one of us lives only by that power, but not recognizing the source, we take the credit unto ourselves for that radiance.

We splatter the window of our consciousness with desires, with likes and dislikes, with anger, jealousy, greed, and all the emotions that human nature is heir to. When we look at most people we don't see God, but we see the window obscured. Occasionally we find someone who, though ordinary, is somehow more beautiful than most. Perhaps he's happier, kinder, more loving, more compassionate than others, and we say he's beautiful. But usually such human beings, even of this type, are limited. They're still capable of losing their sweetness and calmness.

There are very few truly beautiful souls in this relative world. Most of us don't have the opportunity to see a living expression of God, such as a great saint or master who goes beyond all these definitions. We're mistaken if we think of such souls as individuals, because they've lost that sense of individuality. What makes a master beautiful is that you don't see the window anymore, but rather you can see through it. You can see divine love expressed through human love. You can see divine joy expressed through human enthusiasm.

Yet an important thing to bring out is that even though a great master is above human personality, he is at the same time completely human. He helps us to understand that to be completely human is to be more than what we are. It's more accurate to say that we are not *yet* human. We're working at it, because although we have the potential we haven't yet realized that we *are* that Infinite Self.

From that Infinite Consciousness, Jesus manifested a particular personality that was very strong, wise, compassionate, and joyful. He had to have all these wonderful qualities for people of all types to follow him by the thousands. Yet somehow the image has come down to us after two thousand years of somebody who stood there weeping for people's sins and looking sour about everything. You can imagine him as saying, "Lo, I am with you always," like a voice from the tomb. Yet I don't think that many people would follow somebody like that unless they themselves were real "Gloomy Guses."

We're not drawn to people who weep for our sins and the darkness in us, but to those who, in seeing that darkness, still believe in the light behind it. We're drawn to those who offer us hope and promise and who see our potential. That's what Jesus did in reality. He must have been a dynamic person to attract that many people, and he also must have had a great sense of humor to say some of the things he said. There was a lot of courage behind some of his humor.

Once when a crowd were about to stone him, he said, "I've done many good things for you. For which of these good things are you going to stone me?" No coward would say that to an angry mob. If you put yourself in that situation and really visualize it, you cannot think of him as sniveling, "I've done all these good things. Now what are you going to stone me for?" Not at all. There had to be a dynamic will behind him saying, "So I've done all these good things. Now you want to stone me? Go ahead."

He was above anything they could do to him. The Bible says something very interesting here that most people don't notice. It says at that moment he went through the crowd and wasn't even seen. In other words, he dematerialized. So for a few little miracles like that also, we remember him.

Yet the way he expressed the Divine is something that people needed at that particular time. He needed to break an excessive obedience, an obsession you might say, with the law. That's why he said, "The Sabbath was made for man, not man for the Sabbath." That's also why he served people outside the usual class rules of the rabbis, which had become more and more ossified over the centuries. He had exactly the kind of personality that was needed in his day and age.

When we read about great saints and masters, they're usually up in the Himalayas withdrawn from mankind—aloof from it all and untouched. We tend to think that's how a great world savior has to be. Yet that example wouldn't be attractive to everybody. A world savior who has a public mission would inevitably feel the same non-attachment to everything as those souls who have only a small band of disciples around them, but such saviors also come as conquerors. If you look at their lives, you can see that masters who come as world saviors come with great power. Buddha, Krishna, and Jesus all had it. Every one of the great teachers of mankind has been a dynamic person.

So Paramhansa Yogananda came in this role for this age, but as a very modern man. He was very far from being the kind of saint that you would expect when you read books on Yoga and Vedanta with their declarations that nothing exists except the Infinite—*Shivo Ham,* "I am Brahma. I am That." He didn't outwardly show this kind of consciousness. Rather, he was very much aware of things. He was dignified, calm, wise, kind, and compassionate, but at the same time he was a tremendously dynamic person.

When Master was giving lectures across the country as a young man, he would run out onto the lecture platform with his long hair streaming behind him and his robes flapping. The first thing he would say was "How is everybody?" They would all shout back, "Awake and ready!" He had so much power in his expression, and yet also he was so practical. He loved practicality and emphasized it as a particularly American virtue. Master often used to say about finding God, "Eventually, eventually, why not now?" Then he would laughingly say, "That's what I like about the American spirit. They aren't daunted by the immensity of the task."

He came with a radiant, charming personality that out-charmed anybody in Hollywood. He didn't have a "Pepsodent smile," but one that came from the heart and captivated everyone. Often people who met him for the first time later told me they felt his was the most spiritual face they'd ever seen.

In living with him and being in his presence, we saw that everything he did was somehow right for that moment. He could manifest anger if he had to, but he was never truly angry. He could manifest compassion—it was an essential part of his nature. He had all the qualities of a perfect being which the scriptures describe as, "Softer than the flower when compassion is at stake, but stronger than thunder when virtue and justice are at stake." He was such a balance of divine qualities, and had such an ability to react appropriately in the moment that I often found it uncanny.

For one thing, when you think of anybody you're close to, you can bring his or her face to mind. I could never bring his face to my mind until I thought of one of his photographs. I could have seen him five minutes earlier, but still I couldn't remember that face. When I'd meditate, I'd use a photograph because in some uncanny way his face changed all the time. It wasn't the facial structure that changed, but the consciousness behind it. There are many photos of him, but no two are alike.

Often when posed with another person in a photograph, he physically resembled them, because he took on their consciousness. A good example of this is when he was photographed with the president of Mexico, Portes Gil, who was very portly and stout. When Yogananda stood next to him, he looked just like Portes Gil. You might think, "Okay, they looked alike." But then there's another picture of him with Amelita Galli-Curci, the famous opera star, who physically couldn't be more different than Portes Gil. She was delicate, small, and frail, yet somehow in that photograph Yogananda looked like her.

He once told us a story about an artist who was trying to paint Krishna, but finally he had to give up. He pleaded,

"Krishna, please stop changing. I can't capture your face." He had been trying to paint him over a number of days, but each time Krishna looked different because of the needs of that day, the needs of the people he was with, or the divine mood of the moment.

To some extent even we can become unrecognizable to those who know us depending on changes in our consciousness. A friend of mine told me a story that occurred during the riots in Calcutta at the time of the partition of India and Pakistan. There was a mania of murder and destruction that seized the city, and many people were shooting others. Some of the shooting was from fear of being attacked, but some was with blood lust—it was a terrible time.

My friend who was living in Calcutta had to leave his house because his family was beginning to get low on food. He was a hunter, so he took his gun with him for protection. Suddenly he was confronted by the Chief of Police of Calcutta pointing a gun at him, with murderous rage on his face. They had been friends, but at that moment neither could recognize the other because rage had changed his face so much. They stood pointing their guns, and staring at each other. Finally it was as though a mist fell from the Police Chief's face, and he sobbed, "I'm so sorry." He had been crazy because of the madness that had seized that whole city. How is it possible for people to change that much? That's a question in itself, but it can certainly affect their very appearance so that we can't even recognize them.

So Yogananda's appearance changed, too, but in a different way. Because he was so sensitive to others, and there was no ego there, he became the other person in a sense. When he talked to you, he didn't talk from his own experience the way most people do. He talked to your soul according to your particular needs, to who you were, and to the potential that he saw trying to come out. It wasn't as if he got angry if he saw somebody else angry, but he reflected back to you what your higher self would be thinking in response to your anger.

You see, there's something inside each of us that is omniscient. The soul never loses its wisdom or understanding, but the ego gets in the way and becomes the source of our problems. It does this through our desires, our likes and dislikes, and then it obscures our soul's understanding.

You've probably all had experiences of people expressing far greater insight than what is usual for them. This happens especially with children, who sometimes amaze you with their wisdom, because they're a little closer to where we've come from. They haven't yet fully taken on a new personality or a new body with its habits, so the ego doesn't obscure the understanding so much. Therefore something speaks through them that is far wiser than they themselves are. It's not as if they had that wisdom, and yet, it's there for a moment.

Your higher self wouldn't get angry with you if it saw you in a state of anger. We blame ourselves—the soul does not, nor does God. Your soul calmly looks at you, and holds up a mirror to say, "Is this what you want to be? Is this really how you want to act?" If you listen to that inner voice, if you look for that calm expression, you'll suddenly think, "No, I don't want to be that way." That voice is your conscience speaking. Your conscience isn't something bred into you by society—it comes from a much deeper level.

Yogananda did much more than just offer us an example of the ideal man—joyful, loving, compassionate, and understanding. He offered something that is global, rooted in principles, and not just in personality. Master came at a time when the human race is at a crossroads. There are new kinds of understanding welling up in society at large based on breakthroughs in science. At the beginning of this century science discovered that matter is not solid but is actually a vibration of energy.

Theoretically, it's possible to take a loaf of bread, dissolve it back into the energy of which it is a manifestation, and then re-manifest it as a bar of steel. No elements are the same, yet it could be done because all of its atoms are manifestations of cosmic energy. That energy takes on different forms, just as it does in our bodies with the food we eat.

The same energy from food goes to the different body parts to reinforce the nails, hair, eyes, tissues, and organs. Each of these parts is different, and yet they're sustained by the same energy. Then it happens that some higher intelligence revivifies the body—replacing dying cells and adding new ones. The reason new cells exactly replicate the original ones again is that there's a vortex of energy that says, "This is an eye, an ear, toenails, and hair follicles." All of this is conducted, without your awareness, by some higher consciousness that has its root in energy.

Now this is such a radical and revolutionary way of looking at things that we've come to a great crossroads in our thinking. A tension exists between old perspectives, which saw matter only as solid form, and new views, which see the world more as waves of energy. This dichotomy is expressed in many different ways in society today.

One expression of the old view is the thought that we are all separate from each other. Jean-Paul Sartre, the nihilistic French philosopher, said, "To be conscious of someone else is to be conscious of what one is not." This is the perspective of the materialistic mind that sees everything as matter and all things as separate. The conscious, as opposed to superconscious, mind works that way—it analyzes, separates, and tries to see how each thing is different from another. In that process, it splits people, races, and nations apart, and makes all things seem separate.

In our age we see disunity becoming stronger and stronger. I don't understand why it should be, but suddenly we find that people all over the world are thinking in terms of divisions. Countries are trying to secede from other countries or are attacking them. Races are affirming their differences from each other. Women are affirming their differences from men. The blacks are against the whites, and the whites are against the blacks. The French Canadians are against the English Canadians, and so on across the world.

There's less thought of what we can do for our neighbor, and more of what we can get for ourselves. The lawsuits that go on in this country are appalling. Why should people feel that they've got to sue each other for every little thing that happens? Increasingly we see people in confrontation with each other, so that competition has become much more of a way of life than it was even in the days of the robber barons.

Yet there's a new world view coming to the fore which Yogananda came to bring—a view of unity. He brought the world an understanding of the unity of mankind, not based on outward similarities, but based on inner realization that we are all one with God. He brought people together in harmony. There was always in him the ability to see the good side of others, and to find in them something positive. He wasn't dogmatic, or a strict disciplinarian who judged. He didn't judge anybody, but he fired us with enthusiasm to do better.

I heard somebody speak about him once, saying that he insisted on everything being neat, and that he was a great stickler for putting everything in its proper place. Perhaps this person was trying to justify her own harsh attitude towards others who were under her tutelage. Truly Master was the most generous-minded man I've ever known.

I remember once, when I was living at Mt. Washington, when he came unexpectedly to the monks' dining room. The room was in the basement, and we had a very small sink, as well as our shower, there. It was hopeless to keep clean, but let's face it, most of us were young and weren't that concerned with keeping things in order. Well, to face it even further, the dining room was a pigsty. One day it was particularly bad. We hadn't washed up yet—interpret the word "yet" as you choose—and Master came in. I was expecting some sort of a tirade, but he just calmly looked around and said, "It could be worse."

It was so beautiful to see his unceasing kindness. Once he was scolding one of the monks, who afterwards pleadingly said, "But you will forgive me won't you, Master?" He looked astonished and said, "What else can I do?" It didn't occur to him to judge. He was just trying to inspire the monk to do better, and of course he forgave to the extent that there was anything to forgive.

He always looked for that point that brought people together. He was a master of bringing out those things that would help to build a sense of oneness and unity. In that spirit, he urged us somewhere, somehow to build what he called "World Brotherhood Colonies." He envisioned these as places where people would come together to help each other, and to work in cooperation—not competition—with one another. By God's will and grace, I've been able to do that particular work, and Ananda, though it still has a long way to go, is the beginning of the fulfillment of his dream.

The spirit that exists at Ananda is one of selflessness and concern for others first. It's one of serving God and dedicating one's life to Him. I'm so touched by that spirit because this is the kind of community that Yogananda wanted to see happen. I've often told our people, "Our community is not just the people living here. It's our neighbors, our township—it's the whole world." More and more we need to develop in our community that consciousness which sees the veriest stranger as a brother or sister.

Many of our people just do this naturally, and they find that wherever they go, others will help them and do what they can to work with them. Once many years ago I had an interesting experience in this respect. I was going to Europe to visit the Self-Realization Fellowship centers there, and was taking all sorts of things, including a harmonium for the classes I'd be giving. All these things made my baggage quite overweight. The man in front of me at the Pan Am counter also had overweight baggage, but much less than I, and he was being charged for the extra pounds. He was getting more and more angry and was shouting, "I know the president of this company. I demand to see the manager. I'll never fly Pan Am again." The ticket agent almost took pleasure in denying him. At one point the manager came out, but he too was firm that the man had to pay for the excess weight. All he was left with was to splutter, "I will never fly Pan Am again."

I thought, "Brother, I'm the next one up. What do I do now?" So I prayed to Yogananda and Divine Mother and stepped forward just seeing God in the ticket agent. There may have been two things at work here—maybe the agent was just tired of fighting, or maybe it was the result of my trying to see him as my own. In any case, he smiled and said, "Well, what have we got here? Oh, okay." He just passed it all through even though I had a lot more baggage than the other man.

This kind of thing has happened often to me. Another time I recall was once when I was in New Delhi trying to buy a statue of Krishna for our ashram. I found a beautiful marble statue for 400 rupees, which was a large amount of money at that time and more than I could afford. I said to the sales clerk, "This is for an ashram. Would you like to give me a five per cent discount?" He said, "I'm sorry, Sir. This is a government store, and we're not allowed to give discounts."

I thought, "God is in this man, and God in him will listen to this request." Then I looked at him with a very winning smile and said, "Make it 350." This was a twelve per cent discount, not merely five. He looked at me, did a double take, and then said, "All right." So if you reach out to others, not as strangers but as friends, they'll work with you, and somehow it all works beautifully. Many times you'll have made a friend, and sometimes these people become your friends for life.

This spirit of universal friendship is something that Yogananda manifested throughout his life. There's a lovely story about a time that he went into a shop that sold umbrellas and canes. He liked to collect these things because it was one way that he had of keeping his mind down to the body. It's as difficult for a master to keep his mind in the body as it is for us to get out of it.

They have little mannerisms and interests that keep them on the physical plane. Ramakrishna would come out of samadhi and ask for a glass of water or a smoke.

So Yogananda had the hobby of collecting canes and umbrellas. Since he was buying these things for the creation of a museum for the work, he bargained hard and talked the salesman down on every item. Then after the sale was completed, Master turned away from being a bargainer and became a divine friend. He looked around him and thought, "This man is poor." Out of compassion he gave the man far more money than he'd saved in bargaining. The man said, "You're a gentleman, Sir," and he gave him a beautiful umbrella. When Master came home, I remember him saying, "That was such a shabby shop. I think I'll buy him a carpet."

This kind of tenderness toward a complete stranger was something that he showed always because he lived in the consciousness of seeing God in all beings. It's like the story of when a wild tiger in the jungles of India confronted him. By seeing God in that tiger and looking at it with divine love, Master turned it from being ferocious to being gentle. Rather than springing on him, the tiger rolled on the ground, and Master scratched his belly as though he were a pussycat. He would sometimes confront hold-up men and just with a glance of love, just by seeing them as his own, he would totally change their lives.

This vision of seeing the unity in all things doesn't come from putting two disparate things together. It's recognizing that underneath each wave, which seems different in size, shape, and movement, there is the one ocean. So when he saw us, he saw God in all our different forms—God manifest like waves on an ocean, and yet God inside all. In our limited view, we look at things from the outside. It's like looking at the spokes of a wheel from the rim. All the spokes appear to be separate, but when you look at it from the center, you see that they all radiate outward from the hub and are integral parts of it.

In our lives we need to learn this lesson more than anything else. The world is coming more and more to a point where it seems likely to explode into a world war, depression, and gigantic cataclysms. In fact, I remember once in Hollywood Church Master talking about the future and saying with a very strong voice, "You don't know what a *terrible cataclysm* is coming!" It made us quake in our seats.

It seems this world is building itself up to a real period of destruction and suffering, and it's all because we've seen things from the outside. What mankind will gain after this period of cleansing is the understanding that recognizes we're really all one. We're one human race, and we're one in God. Master said that after a period of world upheaval there will be an era of harmony and brotherhood such as never has existed in known history. But the cleansing is upon us, and it's coming because of these two disparate ways of looking at reality—one that sees all things as separate, and the cosmic view that sees all things as one.

The more we can learn to see life as a flow of unity, the more we'll be able to find what we're all looking for— happiness, love, and inner peace. Yogananda came to manifest these qualities. In a very distinct aspect of his mission, he came to bring this vision of unity to everyone—a vision that he manifested in his actions, in his words, and in the example that he set for all of us.

※

Chapter Nine

Karma, Free Will, and Realization

"Don't think that you can master this world—you can't, because the dice are loaded. You can only win the game of life by going back to God, by living in Him."

According to the ancient traditions of India, there are three aspects to spiritual teachings. The first one helps us to understand our *need* to find spiritual truth and to avoid the false perceptions created by the world of the senses. The next tells us how to do it—how to get away from the delusion of the senses and the false expectations that disappoint us in the end. In other words, this aspect shows us *how* to find the Divine. The third, and equally important, aspect describes *what it is we attain* once we unite our souls with God.

Now all of these teachings make one package, you might say, and yet they're all presented separately in Indian philosophy—Shankya, Yoga, and Vedanta. Shankhya talks about the delusive nature of the world. Yoga teaches the techniques and methods for achieving freedom from this world and discovering who we really are. Finally, Vedanta describes that we are, in fact, the Infinite Spirit. As the classic phrase of the Vedanta philosophy puts it, "You are That."

One of the great barriers between our present state of consciousness and the expanded vision of Vedanta is the issue that people have grappled with for millennia: the question of free will. How free are we to change our destiny? What is the meaning of free will?

I had a fascinating experience in this regard many years ago in India. I was taken to a little village in the state of Punjab where there was a segment of a very ancient manuscript, the *Book of Bhrigu,* supposedly written thousands of years ago. I had no way of knowing how old this book was, but one thing about it absolutely fascinated me. It was reputed to be a book of prophecies about the lives of people who would live in the future—people alive today. The pundit who read the book didn't know me, and yet there was a little page which gave my name, Kriyananda; where I was born; and that I was a spiritual teacher. There were many details that were quite accurate—things beyond what this pundit could possibly have known.

It said, for example, that my father had named me "James." Usually people don't know that this is my first name: I was always called by my middle name, "Donald," because there were too many "Jameses" in the area where I grew up. The only way the pundit could have known this would have been to go to the Home Ministry in Rumania, where I was born, and find it there—a very slim chance.

This reading then stated that I was, in fact, born in Rumania, grew up in America, that Yogananda was my guru, and that I later took the name "Kriyananda." It went on to say that I had two brothers, but that no living sister was possible. The page said that one sister would die in my mother's womb. I'd never known that my mother had suffered a miscarriage, but when I got back to America I asked her, and she confirmed this. The pundit also said that I would return to America within two months, and I returned the following month. At the end of my page, there were predictions for my future that, for the most part, have come true.

I took this page to the Indian National Archives Laboratory, and I asked them, "Can you tell how old this page is?" I thought perhaps they could do carbon-14 dating on it to determine the age, but they weren't set up for that process. Then I asked, "Can you at least tell me if it's recent?" They replied, "How recent?" I thought, "Well, I've known this pundit for only two days," so I asked, "A month?" They replied, "Well, if you're thinking of a month, that's easy to tell, because ink will set in a page over a period of time so that it can't be washed away." They took a wet cloth and tried to wipe away some of the writing, but the ink had really set. Finally they told me, "We can't say how old it is, but it's definitely much older than a month."

Then I took the page to the Director of the Archeological Institute and asked him how old it was. He looked at it and said, "It's not very old." This page was, in fact, supposed to be a copy of the original that is reputedly buried somewhere in Tibet. So I asked him, "How old would you say?" He was used to working with very ancient manuscripts from five thousand years ago. So he looked at the page again and said, "It's only about one hundred and fifty years old." Well, that was old enough to be impressive to me.

The interesting thing about this reading was twofold: First, scholars generally think of ancient India as being peopled by a bunch of cowherds. The truth is they must have been extremely advanced in certain areas of knowledge to be able to know such details about people who would live thousands of years in the future. It staggers the imagination.

Second are the philosophical implications: Do we have any free will at all? If someone thousands of years ago could tell that you were going to be born in a certain country at a particular time with a specific name, how much freedom do we really have? In our society we aren't prone to think philosophically as a rule. Our general thought, which is expressed all the time, is that we're perfectly free to do what we want.

But what makes you *want* to do certain things? That's where the rub comes in—you're conditioned to want certain things because you behaved that way in the past. Once when I'd been staying with Yogananda at his desert retreat at Twenty-Nine Palms, I said to him, "I've always wanted to live alone in the desert like this." He replied, "That's because you've done it as a hermit in other lifetimes." I was conditioned to this.

Another interesting aspect of the *Book of Bhrigu* was that it said that in my last life I lived for many years meditating in the desert in Rajasthan. In this life I was born amid greenery and mountains and as a child never even saw a desert. But when I came to Twenty-Nine Palms after meeting Master, I instantly fell in love with it. According to Bhrigu I had had that conditioning in a past life. It just felt like home to me, and I used to say to people, "I feel more at home here than anywhere else I've ever been."

Most of your subconscious memories are well buried, but they manifest themselves in your present life in the form of tendencies, or even in the kind of body that you have. Everything is preordained not by some cosmic destiny, but by your own past actions. What you've done in the past makes you what you are today.

Now the important aspect of this teaching is that if you don't like your present condition, you can change your future by simply behaving differently. Of course, the problem again is how free are you to change? The more you live in ego consciousness, the less free you are. In fact, you don't really have freedom to do anything. That's a gloomy message if you take it by itself, but if you expand on it and realize what the meaning of freedom is, then you come upon a wonderful and very generous truth.

Freedom doesn't mean the ability to do whatever you like. That's impossible. You think, for example, that your body is free to move in whatever way you wish. You're free to jump up in the air, and you're not bound to the earth. But how high can you jump? And how long can you stay in the air? The power of gravity pulls you down to the earth.

You're bound by your society and by the influences that you receive in your life. A child born in America but brought up in India will behave exactly like a Hindu or Moslem child. Some people think it's *only* a matter of social conditioning, but it's deeper than that. In fact, even the kind of body that you have is the result of a choice due to past conditioning. These things aren't decided by some whimsical God, but by the tendencies that you've developed in the past.

What we need to understand is that freedom means the ability to act for your own highest happiness as opposed to the slavery of acting in ways that ultimately bring unhappiness. A young person thinks, "I'm free to do what I want, so I'll get drunk every night." This seems fine at the time, but eventually he'll develop a habit of drunkenness, his will power will be weakened, his mind will become unclear, he'll lose his health, and he may eventually die of liver disease. Bit by bit, it becomes increasingly obvious that he's not free at all, although he has acted in the name of freedom.

You're not free in this body or in this ego. Freedom comes not by being divorced from all conditioning and influences. It means to be influenced by higher truth—not by lower ignorance. You cannot escape the fact that you're a part of God and a part of this great universe. What you need to do is make the best of it. Many people ask God, "Why did you put me in this body? Why have you given me this life?" These aren't useful questions. The fact is, you're here. What you need to ask is, "What can I do about it?"

People accuse God of all kinds of things, and yet God doesn't determine any of it. Many people even lose faith in God, because they see so much suffering in the world, and they assume that He's indifferent. But there's one group of people who never accuse God of anything—that's the people who have found Him. The saints never say, "Well, I know Him now, and did I ever give Him a piece of my mind." Rather they say, "Oh, this whole show was wonderful. All the pains and sicknesses that I went through were worth it, because I learned important lessons. More than anything else, I gained the understanding that my freedom and my fulfillment won't ever be found in this world."

The opinions of others, success in the world, finding the right mate, getting a lot of money—all these are just a fool's paradise. The only thing that we really long for and need in our soul of souls is union with the Infinite and the freedom to live always in joy. The saints who have found God are the ones who are the most positive about the reason for it all.

When you see a child in grade school, you assume that he or she hasn't yet studied calculus. You can't accuse him of being ignorant, for the simple reason that he won't learn calculus until he grows older. We tend to accuse people of certain things and judge them for being dishonest, or selfish, or unkind. What we really ought to do is see that they're in different grades of school, and are learning their appropriate lessons. Once we've learned that our happiness doesn't lie in possessions or pleasures, then no one has to tell us this—we simply know it from our own experiences. Everybody should be given the respect that you give to your own self, respect based on the recognition that behind that ego, God is there trying to come out in each person.

The beauty of the spiritual path is the understanding that the God we're seeking is the same God that's in everybody. Whatever path you follow—or even if you don't follow any path at all—you can't get way from it, because it's the truth of this universe. Whether you're going at it through worldliness or through meditation, you're going somewhere, and that inevitably has to end at the true understanding of who and what you are.

If you go through drunkenness, you get drunk and suffer. Eventually you realize through suffering that that wasn't the way to go. Then maybe in the next life you'll be different, but in one way or another people need the lessons of life. The question is, how long do you want to go on suffering? People don't think of the payment, but only of the immediate reward. They don't realize that for every outer reward, there's going to be some sort of pay-back. There's no free lunch, as they say, no free fulfill-ment in this world.

Why? Because there's a law behind this world of the senses—the law that God is One. In order to create the universe, God had to create the principle of duality. He had to move His consciousness, which is at the heart of all creation, in opposite directions. That's why, as science tells us too, all things exist in a state of vibration. For every plus, there's a minus; for every up, there's a down; for everything there's an opposite state. If you're seeking fulfillment outside yourself, the more that you go in one direction, the more you'll move back again in the opposite direction like a swinging pendulum.

So it is that people get drunk, and the next day they have a hangover. People socialize and party a lot, but at home they feel very lonely. Their fulfillments are always balanced with disappointments. You have heat and cold, light and darkness, pleasure and pain, male and female, and all the various oppositional states that exist in the world. The more you think that you're going to get it together in one area, the more you'll find that it falls apart in another. They used to have a "Fly now—Pay later" plan, and that's what life is like. You fly today, but then you have to pay for it sooner or later. Finally life assumes, as Master put it, "a sense of anguishing monotony," and you begin to think that it's just not worth it.

Gradually some of these lessons sink in, and you know that you don't want to follow those false promises of happiness. For example, in my life I've never wanted to gamble. It's funny that I should feel that way, because in fact the first money I earned in this incarnation was by gambling. When I was six months old and had no control over the situation, my father bet some money at the roulette table and won five hundred dollars. He invested that money in a trust fund for my two brothers and me, and eventually bought stocks for us. The stocks never amounted to very much, but later it helped make Ananda possible.

But throughout my adult life, I've always been suspicious of gambling. When you have a deep-seated understanding about something, Divine Mother helps you, and the Divine law itself cooperates. After I was on the path, I went with my parents once to a party where they were playing bridge for a pittance. This was really pretty harmless, but yet, the thought of gambling was abhorrent to me. At the same time I wanted to be a good son and didn't want to say, "No, I won't play," so I prayed, "Divine Mother, you've got to help me out." I ended up playing, but do you know that my score at the end of the evening was zero? I didn't want to win or lose, so Divine Mother arranged it perfectly. I think the chances of getting a bridge score of zero are infinitesimal.

There are often certain things in life that you may have a natural instinct against. Trust those instincts, and don't think that you have to go against them to prove something to yourself. Smoking cigarettes is a good example of this. When I was in college, someone gave me a cigarette and taught me how to inhale. I tried inhaling, and, of course, like everybody else I became deathly sick. Then I did what a lot of others do if they're stupid enough—I said, "I'm going to lick this thing." This meant proving to myself that I could learn to inhale and not get nauseated. I should have done just the opposite, and said, "I'm going to lick this thing, and then I'm going forget it." But I wasn't smart enough, and it was some time before I could break the smoking habit. That's how this world catches us.

Don't think that you can master this world—you can't, because the dice are loaded. You can only win the game of life by going back to God, by living in Him. Your freedom is basically this: either to accept God or to reject Him. It's the absolute freedom God gives all of us, and although we sometimes have to work hard at it, it's still our inherent soul right.

I used to notice with Yogananda that he would never impose on the free will of other people, even if he saw that what they were bent on doing was something that would bring them harm. He would try to caution them, certainly, but he wouldn't force them. You can't force people to do the right thing or drive it down their throats, but you must give them the freedom to decide for themselves.

The same thing is true with using hypnosis to change people's behavior. Master used to say that hypnosis was a spiritual crime. Yes, people may give up smoking, for example, if they're hypnotized in a particular way, but it will weaken, not strengthen, their will. The subconscious habit of smoking will come out in some other way, because real understanding and change comes from within. You have to give people the freedom to understand according to where they are at the time.

When you give others advice, or when you discipline children, don't try to force them. Allow their understanding to develop from within, and try to draw it out of them. There are times, obviously, when you have to be a little bit more forceful. If a two-year-old is crossing the street against traffic, you have to pull the child back, but you can't make such an absolute rule that the child grows up longing to cross the street into traffic. That's what happens to many children when you try to discipline them with intense emotions and anger. They grow up wanting to do the very thing that you told them they shouldn't, and it's much worse for them in the long run. Let people grow at their own pace and arrive at the right conclusions in their own way. I don't mean, therefore, that you should never say anything, but offer it in such a way to invite, not impose on, their understanding.

So when we consider to what extent we have free will on an outward level, we run up against limitations in all directions. There seems to be an imposition of the Infinite on who we are and what we want. We can find our way out of it only when we give up affirming the ego and stop saying, "I want to be this. I want to be that." So often in our age, perhaps more than in any other, people live in terms of ego fulfillment. They think, "This is who I am. I demand my rights. Others have done me wrong." People today are obsessed with victim consciousness and how badly others have treated them.

Recently I met a psychiatrist from New York, and he asked me what I did. I told him that I try to help people to take responsibility for their own lives, and to learn to stand on their own feet. I said that I encourage them not to blame others or to feel that they're the victims of society. He looked at me and said, "So you're the competition." I said, "Yes, and proud of it."

We've got to learn to take our lumps and become strong. Somebody once asked me, "What is the best yoga posture?" I said, "That posture which teaches you to stand on your own two feet." This is the essence of being a yogi—when you meditate, do it with a straight spine. When you do anything, try to do it because it's your decision, not because somebody told you to. If somebody does tell you to do it, withdraw into yourself and decide if it's something that you can give your will to. If you don't feel your conscience allows you to do it, then don't.

Obedience is good if it's aligned to wisdom, but it's not if it's just blindly obeying a command. I don't know if this is apocryphal or not, but I read that sometimes in convents nuns have been told to plant flowers or vegetables upside down as a sign of their obedience. In other words, they were told to do something that defies common sense in order to learn to obey. If obedience forces you against your will and common sense, then it's doing violence to your nature, and it's not beneficial to your growth. Good obedience is something that will help to support and deepen your understanding. That's why Yogananda said that if you unquestioningly follow someone who isn't enlightened, it can weaken your will. Don't ever give that kind of obedience to anybody unless you come to the point in yourself where you know that person has divine wisdom.

There was one great saint in a Christian monastery who said, "I will do anything for anyone for the sake of strengthening my will power at the expense of my desires, so long as it doesn't go against my conscience." There's another octave of that consciousness—if you make a decision, then be committed to carrying it out. This strengthens your will power. But if everything in you rebels against it, and with a hangdog expression you say, "Well, I guess I've got to do it because he told me to," there's no real benefit for you spiritually.

Learn to be guided more and more from within. This is what Yogananda taught us. Most counselors sit at their desk with their hands folded, look at you wisely, and say, "Now, John, the reason you did this was thus and so." They go on at great length, and there's a lot of talking back and forth. I was quite surprised when I found that Yogananda didn't do much talking at all. If you asked him a question, he would usually answer you with just a phrase or a simple statement, and you'd have to figure out what he meant.

Master did this because he wanted you to rise to the occasion with your own understanding. If you didn't understand from within, what was the use of explaining it? So he would put it in an indirect or hinting way to challenge your own discrimination. Many times I've meditated for years on things that he said to try to understand where he was coming from. The deeper and deeper I go, the more I see how his simple words apply on many different levels.

To give you an understanding of the way he taught, I'll share a story that I've told in my autobiography, *The Path*. Once he stopped and asked me a simple question about astronomy. I used to want to be an astronomer, and at the time I thought perhaps that was why he was asking me the question, which was "What keeps the Earth from flying off into space?" I said, "It's the magnetic pull of the Sun that holds the Earth in its orbit." Then he said, "Well, what keeps the Earth from falling back into the Sun?" I said, "The centrifugal force of our orbit keeps the Earth always pulling in an outward direction." He didn't say anything more, but just smiled. I thought, "How interesting that he wanted this basic astronomical lesson! I hope I've enlightened him."

Months later I suddenly thought, "My God, he wasn't asking about *astronomy*; it was an allegory." It's God's love that keeps us from moving off too far from Him— He's always in our hearts, pulling us back so we can never stray too far. We can never become absolutely evil because God's love in our heart is always there drawing us back to what we really are, and that God is in everybody. But what keeps us from merging back into Him? It's the centrifugal pull of the ego, of our desires, our wish to remain separate, and to get out into the world and do things on our own.

Today we find the world is absorbed more than ever before with the thought of ego and demands to have the freedom to do and be whatever we want. Unfortunately

most people are like children in their understanding—
they get so upset by little things, because they demand
the world be just the way they want it. They have no
mental freedom until they reach the point where they
have some degree of calmness and detachment, where
they can see life as it is and not complain because it isn't
exactly to their liking.

People also try so hard to find freedom by being original in what they do. Original doesn't mean doing something nobody has ever done before—it means doing it
from your point of origin. If you act in that way, whatever you do will be unique, even though others may
have done it before, because *you* are unique in all eterni-
ty. So, to do something originally means to do it as you
feel from within, not from your ego or emotions, but
from your inner inspiration. It may be a very subtle difference, but if you create from within, what you do will
be very different from what anybody else has done
before.

God is Infinite—He can create anew every time. No
two thumbprints or snowflakes are alike. Think of all the
different ways of saying a simple phrase like, "I love
you." The sincerity of the heart makes it unique and
beautiful rather than a trite statement. If there's no sincerity, it's trite immediately, but if it's sincere it will be
reflected in the tone of your voice and the rhythm of
your words. The pitch, the ambience, the moment—
everything somehow makes it uniquely your statement.
It will be fresh every time you say it, as long as you
deeply feel it. Platitudes are only empty words because
they're insincere. If you say something that you deeply
mean, even though the phrase may have been quoted
again and again, somehow it will come to life and
become your own.

We need to live in such a way that we come from inside out, not outside in. Each one has to ask himself, "How am I going to overcome this problem myself? What can I do about it?" The techniques of the ancient science of yoga are universal, and anybody can practice them to improve their life. Master's path offers some of the most central teachings of yoga to help people expand their consciousness towards real freedom.

Yet there's another aspect to the spiritual path that must be mentioned for you to really make progress—you have to make it your own. Your approach to God has to be uniquely yours. How many billions of Christians are there in this world? But there are as many types of Christianity as there are Christians, because each one approaches his prayer differently because of his conditioning. And behind that conditioning, each soul is unique. The influence of conditioning may not produce such great differences in people, but in their soul impulse each one is unique. We need to respect this uniqueness in everybody as well.

Somebody was asking me yesterday, "Why has Ananda succeeded where so many other communities have not?" One of the basic reasons is deep respect for the integrity of every individual. People are free to be themselves. Another key is love for each person, not necessarily as an individual, because some people you like more than others, but as a soul. You can't get away from having personal preferences as a human being, but a devotee should try to train his mind to look deep inside everyone. We should try to see there the perfect soul trying to come out, trying ignorantly mostly, but still trying. The Divine Mother is in all. Learn to love that God in everyone, and it will be possible to love all equally.

You can do this by first loving the Divine in yourself. This can happen only by meditation and feeling the presence of God within. Then you're filled with love, and that love spills over until you feel it for everyone without even trying. You find yourself automatically wanting to bless even people you pass in the streets, especially if they look unhappy, or tense, or caught up in worldly ambitions. You see that that's not really who they are.

Treat people as they really are, and you will find they tend to respond accordingly. They may think they're getting this expanded self-awareness from you, but what they're actually getting is the sudden recognition of who they really are. This is what was so wonderful living with Yogananda—he gave us faith in our own potential. He helped us to recognize who and what we are. We wouldn't say, "Ah, this is what I am. I've got a new definition." But somehow we would recognize in him our own potential for love, for kindness, for joy, and we would begin to feel that it was the only thing about us that was worthwhile.

There's a story about a waiter who served Master in the dining car of a train when he was traveling back and forth across the country during his "lecture campaigns." The waiter was very enthusiastic about serving him, but one day the tables he waited on were full, so Yogananda was placed at another table. Though he didn't even know who Yogananda was, the man was crushed that he couldn't serve this complete stranger. Later he sought out Yogananda in the passenger compartment, and asked him, "What have you got that I want?" Master looked at him deeply and blessed him; the man's life was changed.

What you need to do is show people not your own goodness—that's nothing, that's between you and God—but help everybody get at least a glimmer of their own potential. This is how we can serve other people, much more than helping the poor or the sick. All of these things are good in themselves, but the greatest thing we can do is to help people develop faith in themselves.

I remember when I was in college, a cousin of mine wrote me a letter saying she wanted to become a doctor. I wrote back and said, "That's a very laudable ambition. But it made me realize that what I want to do with my life isn't to take sick people and make them well, because I see that even when they're well they're not happy. I want to spend my life helping well people to become better, to become really well."

I didn't yet fully know what that meant, but I knew that it was the most important thing to do for other people—to help them find inspiration in their life. This personality thing is a great and colossal delusion. Somebody becomes a teacher and suddenly everybody's looking up to him, and he starts thinking, "I'm pretty good." Who are we really? Nothing. When we look at who we are as personalities, we're like dust in the wind.

There's nothing that a human being can do that's really very important. I've been reading some books written back at the beginning of the century which talk about all these important people. Today none of them are known anymore—they're all forgotten names. You can't do anything that's really important in the eyes of the Infinite, except claim your true importance—oneness with Him. Meditate and claim your divine kinship with God. Once you have that, you'll know that you're a master in this world. You'll know that you're an emperor because you're in control, not of other people, but of your own thoughts and impulses.

Be a lion of self-control and centeredness. Live from your center, and you'll find that wherever you go, you have the freedom to make the right decisions. What other people think and do just won't matter to you. If you do what's right in your eyes, and in the eyes of God within, you can never go wrong.

So claim this freedom within, as a child of God, to go toward Him. You won't have freedom in any other way except by turning every action toward the Divine. Offer everything that you do to Him. There's nothing too little to be given to God. In the *Bhagavad Gita*, it says, "Whoever offers Me even a leaf or a flower, I accept that devotion, and I Myself come to receive it." The more you hold to that faith, the more you'll see it becoming real in your life, and you'll know the only true freedom—oneness with God.

Chapter Ten

The Light of Superconsciousness— The Dawn of a New Age

"The realization will come that the power to understand any subject comes from inside, not from absorbing increasing amounts of external data. Real understanding doesn't depend on more and more information, getting Ph.D. after Ph.D., and specializing in this and that until your brain practically explodes with all that weight of information."

Yogananda said that when the world entered the Dark Age of Kali Yuga some 2600 years ago, it became incapable of a broad and balanced perspective. To help mankind survive into a more enlightened age, the Divine plan at that time was that different nations would specialize in different areas of human development. So it was ordained that the East would concentrate on the inner life, and the West would concentrate on the outer one. Yogananda was born in 1893, but the beginning of his mission was actually long before that. It began, in a sense, with this separation between East and West in Kali Yuga, and came to the fore with the dawning of Dwapara Yuga, when it was time to bring this separation to an end. Today we have reached a sufficient level of understanding where we can begin to incorporate the inner and outer life, and see them as one.

It's interesting, in light of what Yogananda said about this conscious divergence of East and West, that toward the end of the first millennium, Pope Leo IX said he'd received a vision that corroborated this thought. He said that he was shown that the Church in the West was to concentrate on the outer religion, whereas in the East the focus was to be on the search for the inner Self. Further he was told that the time would come in the future when these two separate paths would once again unite.

Yogananda said that the avatar who was responsible for the spiritual growth and development of the East was Babaji, that is Krishna in the form of Babaji, and for the West it was Jesus Christ. When Babaji was living in the Himalayas about 1860, Jesus Christ appeared to him and said, "What has happened to my church? It has gotten away from the teaching of communion with God. Though there are still a few souls who commune with Him, by and large the church concentrates on outward activities and ceremonies. Let us send someone to the West to bring back the knowledge of the inner Self and its relationship with God." Thus Yogananda's guru, Sri Yukteswar, said that was why Yogananda was born and sent to him for training—to bring the teachings of Kriya Yoga and inner communion to the West.

It's interesting to note that England went to India and brought the knowledge of the West there, because India needed to balance its inward life with the outward efficiency of the West. Another interesting sidelight on history is that England is the oldest continuous government in the world, the second being our own country. England's government dates back to the conquest of William the Conqueror, who brought England to a level of security, stability, and legal organization that made it possible for it to survive the death of medieval society and continue on into the modern age.

Part of what William did was to change the typical medieval practice of having the serfs and lesser nobles pledge their loyalty first to their own local baron rather than to the king. Prior to William's reign, if a baron rose in rebellion against the king, all his serfs and nobles had to follow him. William introduced the system of pledging loyalty first to the king, and with that method he united the whole kingdom. This enabled England to endure when other countries fell apart into warring duchies.

When you look at the history of Italy, for example, you see that it was a constant cycle of city-states warring with each other. If you go there, you see the walls that surrounded those towns actually encircled quite a small area. But such was the course of history in those days that even the battle of a few people became a major historical event. The concept of a unified nation didn't really exist then, but rather there were dispersed populations who agreed in some vague way to speak a similar language. The people of Italy actually only became Italians at heart when they won the World Cup a few years ago. Before that they were all citizens of their own cities—*Napolitani, Milanesi, Fiorentini,* and so on.

To return to our central theme, God and the great masters ordained Yogananda's mission, and it was Jesus who actually sent him. This is why he often had visions of Jesus, because his mission was to bring back the original teachings of Christ and the original yoga of Krishna, and to show the oneness of those two scriptures. This is also why I read from the Bible and the *Bhagavad Gita* at our Sunday Services, and why I wrote the book, *Rays of the Same Light,* to compare parallel passages in them.

In January 1894 Sri Yukteswar went to the *Kumbha Mela,* the great spiritual gathering that takes place every twelve years near Allahabad, India. There he met Babaji, and at that meeting Babaji told him to write a book that would interpret these two scriptures and show how they are one. Within the year Sri Yukteswar completed this book, which he called *The Holy Science*. This is a book destined for the ages, and like many such books, it's pretty hard to follow in the particular age you're living in. It's a very deep book that goes to the heart of Yoga, Vedanta, the divine teachings, and the inner life. It interprets the scriptures in ways that the rational mind can't easily follow—it takes the intuitive, superconsciousness to be able to see how profound this commentary is.

Yogananda came to bring these teachings out of the recondite, mystical atmosphere of caves and ashrams and into the marketplace. His mission, and that of his whole line of gurus, was to bring these teachings to people everywhere. Those of you who have read *Autobiography of a Yogi* will remember when Lahiri Mahasaya met Babaji in the Himalayas. Babaji said, "Bestow the Kriya key only on qualified chelas. He who vows to sacrifice all in the quest of the Divine is fit to unravel the final mysteries of life through the science of meditation."

Lahiri Mahasaya pleaded, "I pray that you permit me to communicate Kriya to all seekers, even though at first they cannot vow themselves to complete inner renunciation." Babaji replied, "Be it so. The divine wish has been expressed through you. Give Kriya to all who humbly ask for help."

So it was that Lahiri Mahasaya, a householder, brought this technique to monks, householders, and people everywhere. Through him, it was given to Sri Yukteswar, who was first a householder and then a monk. Then he, in his turn, gave it to Yogananda who was completely a monk. In this way they showed that these great masters cannot be separated from each other, but that they're all part of the line which we must see as a continuum to get a complete picture of what any one of their teachings is all about.

People today who exclusively follow Lahiri Mahasaya's line criticize Yogananda for starting an organization. They say Lahiri Mahasaya was against organizations, but, frankly, all masters are against them. They don't have any use for the claim that an organization can teach a truth and crystallize it so that it can be better disseminated. They understand that truth is something that must be realized within and then passed from individual to individual.

Yet they also understand the need for organization—it's a necessary evil, you might say, because without an organization of some kind the teaching would die out. It would very soon slip back into being a hidden teaching or a mystery school. It needs to be brought out into the marketplace, and thus the need for organization. Thus also is the need for uniting East and West, because the East is pretty hopeless when it comes to organizing anything.

I remember an incident typical of this when I was invited by the Indian students at California Medical College in San Francisco to give a slide show on India. They told me they'd have a screen and projector, and would have everything all set up for me—all I had to do was bring the slides. I brought the slides—but there was no screen. So people were running around trying to find a screen, which they finally found and set up, but then the projector didn't work. Finally they found a projector that worked, but I just couldn't help laughing, because it was so Indian.

I love India, but when it comes to getting things done efficiently, they have a lot to learn. They've had to learn our ways of doing things, and we've had to learn their ways. Neither way is right or wrong. Each is charming in its own way, but to make this world function in Dwapara Yuga, an age of energy and greater enlightenment, we need a balance of both.

To help achieve this balance, Yogananda said that many Indians who are being born today are reincarnations of Westerners, and, more particularly, of Americans. If you go to Bombay, or cities where India is really in the Twentieth Century, the people you see look just like Wall St. stockbrokers—brown-skinned, but nevertheless, they've got all the attitudes, the consciousness, and mannerisms of Westerners. They've brought that into Indian bodies. When you look around at the ashrams in America, you could swear that you were looking at Indians with white skin.

When I lectured at Cultural Integration Fellowship in San Francisco, California, people used to say that Dr. Chaudhuri, the director, was a Westerner in an Indian body, and that I was an Indian in a Western body. I don't really think that this was so, but he was very much aware of Western ways of doing things, as well as being deeply steeped in Indian teachings and philosophy. He wasn't a businessman type of Westerner in his consciousness at all, but he was efficient. I have had a hard time all my life persuading myself that I'm really an American, because the Western way of looking at things is not natural for me. My natural way is more Indian, and I feel at home there.

This is all a part of the divine process of bringing the East and West together. Master prophesied that in the future India and America would unite, not politically, but spiritually, to lead the world on the path of balanced living—of inward and outward efficiency. Part of his mission was to bring that particular genius of India—the concentration of the mind, the ability to awaken the inner energies, and the expansion of consciousness—to help Westerners see that this is the next step in our unfoldment.

How much farther can we really go in an outward way? Scientists tell us that the universe is composed of a hundred billion galaxies. Next year they'll discover that it's not one hundred, but two hundred billion. What's the difference? We can't even count to one billion. You read predictions about the future, and they're all about the different kinds of gadgets and inventions that people are going to develop.

We may have wonderful things, but that's not going to give us comfort, satisfaction, or what we're really look-ing for. The more complex our lives become, the more it drains our energy. We find ourselves losing our peace of mind. We think that once we've got a television set in the bedroom, the bathroom, the laundry room, the kitchen, and one in the dining room, then we'll be happy. But once you get these things, you begin to think, "Am I happier?" and you have to admit, "No, I'm not."

Someone once asked the multimillionaire, Howard Hughes, one of the richest men in the world, if he was happy. This was just a few weeks before he died, and he said, "No, I can't say I'm happy." The very tone of his voice was full of misery, suffering, and disillusionment. How can you not be disillusioned when you thought that your happiness lay in one direction, and suddenly, like a stream going into the desert, it just evaporates?

How can we look forward to a future with more and more material complexity and satiety? I read a fascinating book called *Looking Backward* by Edward Bellamy, which was written in 1890. It's about time travel and what the future will be like. The hero is sent into the future and finds all sorts of wonderful things there, such as the ability to pipe beautiful music into the home at any hour of the day. To him this was the *summum bonum* of human seeking. Yet everyone here today probably has that capability in the form of radio, tapes, or CDs, and are we happier? I can't say that we are.

Look, too, at the incredible overload of information that we're faced with today. People are becoming so specialized in their fields that they aren't able to get an overall understanding of their profession. I know a doctor who's not only a heart specialist, but he only does one type of heart surgery. A friend of mine, who is also a doctor, told me that it's nearly impossible to keep up with all the medical manuals and periodicals describing new discoveries. They're trying to deal with the problem by putting all the new information on computer, but the human brain can only absorb so much data.

If we keep going in that direction, I can imagine that in a hundred years from now people are going to feel increasingly incompetent, because we'll become overwhelmed with all this detail. But the answer to it, as far as I can see, will be quite unexpected—it will be a greater simplification. The realization will come that the power to understand any subject comes from inside, not from absorbing increasing amounts of external data. Real understanding doesn't depend on more and more outward information, getting Ph.D. after Ph.D., and specializing in this and that until your brain practically explodes with all that weight of information. It will come from getting back to the pristine quality of the brain and consciousness, getting back to the simplicity of who we are.

The time has come, in fact it's been moving towards us for many years now like a great wave, to realize that the future direction of our development is to emphasize the inner world, the inner man. We've focused too much on the world outside, and now we've got to start discovering who we really are and how we fit into the larger picture.

Yogananda came with a perfect blend of the qualities of East and West. His life perfectly embodied the teachings of the East, yet he loved the practicality and efficiency of the West. He wasn't one of these world-renouncing yogis who have nothing to do with anything modern. On the contrary, he had many little gadgets, which he greatly enjoyed, and he even invented things.

Even in his dress, he brought the two cultures together. He only wore orange robes on ceremonial occasions, but usually wore a business suit and a scarf. He said, "I like Western dress because it's so much more efficient than the Eastern garb." In fact, by watching his example we can see how we can blend East and West perfectly in our own lives, because the ideal person will be a balance of the two. The ideal person will be neither man nor woman, Easterner or Westerner, but a blend of everything, with the heart quality and reason in balance.

Master was such a remarkable blend of masculine and feminine qualities. He had a very strong will, but he also prayed to God as the Divine Mother. Many people would say, "He looks like a mother." I remember an incident that happened right after his *mahasamadhi* when all the monks went into his room for a last view of his body. It was a very moving occasion, because he was our father, mother, friend—he was everything to us. But I was especially touched by one of the monks who, when he came up to the bed to make his prostrations to him, said with great fervor, "Mother!" That's what he was to us in a very real sense—our Divine Mother.

We vitally need that Mother concept of God in the West now. We need the balance of reason and feeling, because reason is an important tool, but not if it's to the exclusion of everything else. The tendency of reason is to analyze, to separate, to break up the jigsaw puzzle into lots of little pieces, and then see how they fit together. But the feeling quality, when it's calm and intuitive, sees a flow in life and how things relate to one another.

Women who go more by feeling have this quality more naturally. The reason women are becoming so outspoken today is that deep within themselves they recognize the need for this balance. They recognize that the masculine tendency toward reason has gone too far, and everything's getting off balance because of this. I believe that what will finally come out of the feminist movement is that there will be greater mutual respect and appreciation for both masculine and feminine energy. I think marriage should be based on such mutual appreciation, not just recognition, of differences, because when both aspects work together harmoniously, then each individual grows in depth and realization of their potential.

I've always had a deep-seated suspicion of too much reason, because I find that it can be used to justify anything. I've used it myself in that way just for fun. But ultimately how do you know what is right? It's only when you come back to your feeling, and feel within whether something's right or wrong that you know for sure. In the work that I've done in developing Ananda, it's not been enough for me to see that a certain direction is reasonable to follow. I need to feel it, and I won't take even a step until I do. After that you can bring reason into the picture, and ask if there's anything more to consider in making a decision.

Yogananda said that feeling should be kept in a state of reason. When you have a feeling, don't let it be emotional, because many times that can fool you. Offer it up to reason, which is centered at the point between the eyebrows, whereas feeling is centered in the heart. Offer your heart's feelings up to the spiritual eye and ask, "Is this right?" Then let the spiritual eye and the intellect check with the heart and see if the feeling still rings true. When the two are in harmony, then you have the perfect relationship in yourself. This also produces the perfect relation between men and women and the perfect blend of a human being, who is only half a person until he incorporates into himself his own opposite. That opposite isn't really outside you—it's within you, because we are both feeling and reason.

Yogananda came also to show that religion is practical and to help people see that it's something that you can use in your daily life. This is the ancient tradition even in India, but one that's been lost sight of. The Vedas are really multidimensional, and were intended to improve every aspect of life.

Master brought this practical aspect of religion to light in the West by helping us to see that our minds are very powerful. He said, for example, that when you want something very strongly, you'd better be sure that it's the right thing, because it will come to you—*and* it may nip you in the heel. There's a story Sri Yukteswar told of a man who was sufficiently developed in yoga to have great mental power. He was told that there was a special tree that had a divine blessing, a wish-fulfilling tree.

When you sat under this tree, if you had yogic power, you could instantly materialize whatever you wanted. He began seeking this tree, and after many years he finally found it. At long last he sat down under the tree, and what did he wish for? Samadhi? No, he was a worldly kind of yogi, so he wished for a palace, and it immediately appeared. Then he wished that it be filled with courtiers and beautiful furnishings, and immediately it was so. He thought, "This is just wonderful. I am absolutely contented." As he toured around all the rooms, he was thrilled with their beauty and comfort.

Then he came downstairs to the first floor, and found himself in an empty room. There was nobody there, and the window was wide open. Because the palace was, in fact, out in the jungle, he could hear a tiger roaring not very far away. The thought came to him, "Oh, I hope that tiger doesn't jump through this window. There are no guards in this room to protect me, and the tiger might eat me." He had forgotten that he was sitting under a wish-fulfilling tree, and the tiger did, in fact, jump through the window and eat him.

Sri Yukteswar told this story as an illustration that you have to use your mind wisely, because any wish that you put out will sooner or later come to you. If you wish it strongly, it will come sooner, but even if it comes later, it will still come. So as you develop your mental power, you must also develop discrimination. Yogananda said, "Use your spiritual power wisely." Use it to help people, not for self-aggrandizement. Don't seek wealth, pleasure, and all the things that people normally want in the world. Seek to serve God in others.

Master was able to bring tremendous will power into his outward activities to show us how to accomplish things. When he wanted to purchase Mt. Washington for his headquarters, the owners were asking $45,000 for it. At that time this was a lot more money than it is now— probably more like one million dollars today. Somebody said to him, "It will take you twenty years to get that much money." Yogananda's reply was, "Twenty years for those who think twenty years, twenty months for those who think twenty months, and three months for those who think three months." And he got the money in three months.

This was an illustration that he used to help us understand that we shouldn't be afraid to use our will power for good things, but we must first attune it to the Divine. Always ask God, "Is this what you want? Is this the direction you want me to go?" In this way, we can align our will with wisdom, because true yogis are people of great will power.

Another thing that Yogananda came to teach is that spirituality is dynamic and powerful, not like the common concept of Jesus Christ: "Gentle Jesus, meek and mild." They portray Christ as smiling in a soupy way and sighing for our sins, but he, like every true master, was a person of great power. Master taught how to develop this power in order to realize that religion is for the strong, not for the weak.

He told us one of the basic attitudes that he came to promote in the West was the understanding which is found in the *Bhagavad Gita*—that this world is not going to give us what we're looking for. As long as we're living in it, we should live right. Hence, we shouldn't renounce it, deny it, or denounce it. We should live efficiently and constructively, but we should always understand that reality is within, and that ultimately the goal of life is to find our relationship with God.

The essence of spirituality is renunciation, but not necessarily formal or outward renunciation in the sense that everybody's got to join a monastery. Today we find the monasteries are decimated, and you see the greatest monasteries in Italy with only four or five old monks in their eighties living there. It seems to be the Divine plan for now that people get married and live their renunciation in a more balanced outward way in order to bring about this unity of East and West.

At Ananda we've based our lives on renunciation, but generally it's householder renunciation. It's the idea that we don't own anything for ourselves—we own it for God. We don't work for ourselves—we work for God. We don't work to satisfy our own desires—we work to satisfy God's will. In this way, you can live in the world as an ordinary person with a job and family, but in your daily life, you put God first and meditate morning and evening. While you work, tell yourself constantly, "I'm doing this for you, Lord, for you, Divine Mother. I'm serving through my actions, through my duties and responsibilities, but they aren't mine."

This attitude is essential. Often you see New Age religions, many of which are actually inspired by the teachings of Yogananda, use these teachings to help people become wealthy or to manifest their desires. They keep talking about how if you think right, everything will go your way. I don't know how many times people have told me that because of their spiritual practices, when they drive downtown a parking place opens up for them. They talk about these marvelous things that have happened, and in fact, they do. I could tell a hundred stories like that, but that's not what it's all about, so don't put too much emphasis on it.

Rather remember that this world is all just a dream. Yogananda was constantly emphasizing to us the need to disengage ourselves from both the successes and failures of this world. The ultimate aim of life is to finally withdraw from all of it and to merge into the Infinite—it's not to create a better world that we can all live in happily ever after. If you see your child playing in a mud puddle, you don't try to pretty up the mud puddle. You try to take him out of the mess altogether.

So the real mission of the masters that Yogananda brought to the West was not to tell us how to get a comfortable, successful, and prosperous life, but to show us how to use those things in order to further our inner life. Why should we have to consider them at all? Because when people are poor, they're too busy worrying about where their next meal is coming from to think about God. In the ashrams in India, I almost never saw somebody from the poorer classes. It was almost always people who were from middle class or well-to-do families that came. Why? Because they had enough material comfort to know that's not what they wanted.

In Yogananda's interpretations of the *Bhagavad Gita*, he talks about the statement that even if you fall from yoga, you'll be reborn in a well-to-do home where you can quickly satisfy your desires. In other words, to be born into a good home is often the sign, though by no means an infallible one, of some spiritual leaning. Nonetheless, when people are spiritually inclined, they'll be given the opportunity to fulfill their desires. Even if they've fallen from the path, the fact that they've tried a little bit is a sign of good karma. In their next life, they'll be given an opportunity to work out that karma more quickly, and thus renew their spiritual efforts without much delay.

The *Bhagavad Gita* also talks about the fact that to have prosperity isn't wrong. "Do your duty in the world," is Krishna's counsel to Arjuna, "but at the same time, never forget who you really are." Ultimately we must live for that higher truth. The more determined and dedicated we are, the more quickly we'll burn away all other desires until all that remains is the desire for God.

We all must deal with egoic desires until our karma is perfectly balanced, but the best way to satisfy your desires is to offer them to God. Everything that you give to Him will come back to you in one way or another— don't worry about that. The more you live in God, the more you'll find that your fulfillment is in Him, not in anything outward.

Yogananda taught us to restrain our senses, involvements, and desires, and to live more and more for God. I've often smiled at the way the great masters describe the path of moderation, because to a worldly person moderation means to meditate five minutes a day, and then go out and have a good time. To a master the path of moderation means not to meditate twenty-four hours a day, but to get a little sleep also. They're looking at moderation in a very different way, and are saying, "Don't be such a fanatic, because then you'll get all tense and strained." But they're also saying, "Be as dedicated as you can be," because the more you give yourself up to God, the more you'll find a wonderful freedom coming that nothing can compare to.

Yogananda gave us another approach to spiritual growth that wasn't an absolute teaching but a directional one: Wherever you are right now, try to be better. Wherever you are tomorrow, try to be better than that. Everyday meditate a little more deeply than the day before. Keep trying, but remember that growth isn't a sudden thing—it's a gradual process. You continue to grow until suddenly you find all your inner obstacles have fallen away.

He used to say, "Don't put yourself down when you make a mistake." The other day somebody came to me weeping because, as she said, "I've tried so hard to overcome my anger, but I just can't seem to get anywhere. Every time I think I've got it, then I blow it again." I said, "Look, it's happening much less frequently, isn't it?" She said, "Well, yes." I replied, "Isn't that all you can ask, that you keep trying and that it get better? Finally it will just go."

It's like that man who took Kriya Yoga initiation, even though he couldn't overcome his drinking problem. People said to him, "How can you take initiation into a sacred technique when you can't control your drinking?" He said, "Well, I can't help the drinking, but at least I *can* do Kriya and keep trying." He told me he practiced Kriya with a glass of whiskey in one hand and his Kriya beads in the other. Every now and then, he'd take a little drink and go on doing his Kriyas. You might say, "That's wrong. That shouldn't be," but he was going in the right direction and was trying. The day finally came when he thought, "I'm getting much more out of Kriya than I am out of drinking," and he put the bottle away and never looked at it again.

I had a similar experience when I tried to give up smoking. I had taken it up in college, and though I wanted to give up the habit, it was very difficult to do. I found myself like Mark Twain, who said, "Smoking is the easiest habit in the world to give up. I've done it a thousand times." It was like that for me—I'd repeatedly give it up, but then I'd go back to it. Fortunately I had the good karma to understand how to work on these things. Instead of saying, "I've failed," every time I went back to smoking, I would say, "Well, I haven't *yet* succeeded." It's like a painter—if he gets a line wrong, he says, "I didn't get that quite right. Let me try again."

After a year of this constant affirmation of potential success, "I haven't yet succeeded," I came to the point one night when I just knew that I was never going to smoke again. I told my roommate that I was giving up smoking, and he laughingly said, "Oh yeah, I've heard that one before," but after that night I was never even tempted to smoke again.

"Don't worry about your faults," Yogananda used to say, "but just keep trying." Worry only about this—that you love God enough. God excuses many things when you love Him, and not very much when you don't. Don't think you can get out of delusion just by following the law. Above all else, you must worship Him, love Him, and love the Divine Mother as Her child. Say to Her, "Naughty or good, Mother, I am your own." Then you will find the inner freedom that you've been seeking.

Don't worry about how many times you feel tempted to give up your spiritual search and go back to a worldly life. As long as you keep one thing: If your love for God is strong enough, everything else bit by bit will vanish. As Yogananda said, "God doesn't watch your faults. He just watches whether you love Him." Bit by bit you'll find that you can look back and say, "How I've changed! I don't recognize that old person anymore. It's no longer me."

Don't ever, *ever* say, "I've failed. I give up." If you do, you're lost for this lifetime, and maybe for others as well. If you keep on trying, even at death's door, you will be able to conquer and free yourself from what looked like massive obstacles that were facing you.

Yogananda taught in a marvelous way for people of this day and age, a way that directly answers the problems that are paramount in our lives today—cynicism, doubt, confusion, and despair. His message was one of hope, strength, and practicality. He taught us not to say, "Why is it so?" but "What can I do about it?" Don't think, "If only I were somebody else. If only the situation were different. If only. . . ." All these thoughts are about the wonderful world of might-have-been.

Be practical. Accept the world as it is, and accept yourself as you are. These are the tools you've got to work with. Don't say, "If only I were like St. John of the Cross or St. Francis." If you knew anything about their lives, you'd realize they had their troubles too, but they had the strength, the faith, and the devotion to keep trying.

Be like that—be a hero for God. I think one of the greatest things that Yogananda came to bring was an example of a spiritual hero—bloodied, but unbowed. How often he used that expression! I'm sure he was deeply hurt by the people who betrayed him. How could he not be hurt? He had a tender heart. But at the same time, he said, "It's my joy to be hurt. It's my joy to suffer these difficulties, because it's one more gift I can give God."

When you can develop that attitude, then you find such sweetness coming upon you that no matter what people say or do to hurt you, to destroy you, or to work against what you're trying to do, you just feel blessed by God, because it's all for Him. If at the end of life, you can reach that point of understanding where you realize that success isn't determined by what you've accomplished but by having an attitude of total surrender to the Divine, then you've won the battle.

I've meditated on Yogananda's life for nearly fifty years now, and still I don't feel I've begun to plumb the first layer of the greatness that he manifested. As I study his life, I see how varied it was, and how pertinent it was to every phase of human existence in a very practical way. Yet at the same time his emphasis was always to bring people back to who we really are, what we really want out of life, and why we are here. He never compromised that ideal.

Yogananda was a harbinger sent by God to help us lift our eyes to the dawn of a new age of divine realization. Everything he taught—devotion to God as Divine Mother, the use of will power and energy, Kriya Yoga, cooperative communities, balancing Eastern religion with Western efficiency—are the hallmarks of a new expression of spirituality for Dwapara Yuga. Above all, he showed us that we are here to live for God alone, and we will never be satisfied until we have found that Infinite joy and made it our own. Having dedicated my life to trying to understand and share his teachings with others, I deeply believe that his mission was one of global unity, and that he brought people everywhere that ray of hope and clarity that will bring about a new age of divine awakening.

Dates and Places for Each of the Talks:

Chapter 1 – *The Cycles of Time—Keys to Planetary Evolution* – January 9, 1996 at Ananda Village, Nevada City, California.

Chapter 2 – *Worshipping God as Divine Mother* – January 12, 1996 at New Renaissance Bookstore in Portland, Oregon.

Chapter 3 – *A Tribute to Paramhansa Yogananda* – January 13, 1996 at Ananda Church in Portland, Oregon.

Chapter 4 – *Kriya Yoga—The Universal Science* – January 14, 1996 at East West Bookshop in Seattle, Washington.

Chapter 5 – *Paramhansa Yogananda—The Power of Divine Love* – January 15, 1996 in Ananda Church of Seattle, Washington.

Chapter 6 – *Ananda Village—How It Was Started, and Why* – January 16, 1996 at Ananda Community in Seattle, Washington.

Chapter 7 – *How to be a True Disciple* – January 24, 1996 at Ananda Church in Seattle, Washington.

Chapter 8 – *A Cosmic Vision of Unity* – January 25, 1996 in Sacramento, California.

Chapter 9 – *Karma, Free Will, and Realization* –
January 28, 1996 for Sunday Service at Ananda Church
in Palo Alto, California.

Chapter 10 – *The Light of Superconsciousness—The Dawn
of a New Age* – January 28, 1996 for an evening lecture
in Palo Alto, California.

Glossary

Autobiography of a Yogi ~ A classic spiritual autobiography by Paramhansa Yogananda, the first yoga master of India whose mission it was to live and teach in the West.

Babaji ~ The guru of Lahiri Mahasaya. He is a deathless avatar living in the Himalayas. Stories of his life are included in *Autobiography of a Yogi*.

Bhagavad Gita ~ "Song of the Lord." The Hindu Bible which includes the sacred sayings of Lord Krishna, compiled millenniums ago by the sage Byasa.

Day of Brahma ~ The period of time in which God has manifested creation.

Dwapara Yuga ~ The second of a cycle of four ages outlined in Hindu texts and the age in which we are presently living.

Energization Exercises ~ A system of exercises developed by Yogananda to recharge the body at will and to develop divine awareness in its most subtle aspects.

Guru ~ Spiritual teacher and guide.

Gyana, Gyanic ~ "Wisdom." A gyana yogi practices wisdom as a path to God.

The Hollywood Church ~ A Self-Realization Fellowship church located in Hollywood.

Kali Yuga ~ The Dark Age. The fourth of a cycle of four ages outlined in Hindu texts.

Karma ~ "Action or fate." The effects of past thoughts and actions from this or previous lifetimes.

Kriya Yoga ~ A meditation technique using mental focusing and breath control; the highest meditation technique taught by Paramhansa Yogananda.

Lahiri Mahasaya ~ The guru of Sri Yukteswar, Lahiri was a great Kriya Yoga master and a householder monastic.

Mahasamadhi ~ "Great" samadhi. The final meditation during which a perfected master merges into cosmic consciousness and leaves his physical body.

Master ~ A name of respect for one's guru, who is master of himself. In this book "Master" refers to Paramhansa Yogananda.

Maya ~ Cosmic delusion.

Mt. Washington ~ The headquarters of Self-Realization Fellowship located in Los Angeles.

Night of Brahma ~ The period of time in which God withdraws outward creation back into Spirit.

Patanjali ~ The foremost ancient exponent of yoga.

Rubaiyat of Omar Khayyam ~ A famous poem written by Omar Khayyam, a highly advanced mystic and spiritual teacher. The quatrains express in deep allegory the soul's romance with God.

Samadhi ~ A superconscious state of ecstasy in which the yogi perceives the identity of soul and Spirit. The highest step on the Eightfold Path of Yoga as outlined by Patanjali.

Self-realization ~ Defined by Paramhansa Yogananda: "The knowing – in body, mind, and soul – that we are one with the omnipresence of God."

Self-Realization Fellowship (SRF) ~ The organization founded by Paramhansa Yogananda based in Los Angeles.

Sri Yukteswar ~ Yogananda's guru; a great "gyana yogi" avatar. He was also a Vedic astrologer and author of *The Holy Science.*

St. Augustine ~ A great Christian saint known as the "Saint of the Intellect." His inspiration has touched civilization for over 1500 years.

Vedas ~ The most ancient scriptures of India.

Yogananda ~ Paramhansa Yogananda, "Incarnation of Love." The guru of Swami Kriyananda and the author of *Autobiography of a Yogi.*

Yuga ~ "Great eons." A cycle or subperiod of creation.

About the Author and the Editor

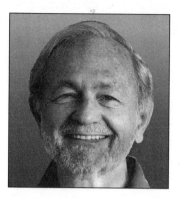

J. Donald Walters is a direct disciple of Paramhansa Yogananda. After receiving instruction from Yogananda to spend his life writing and lecturing, Walters has dedicated the last 50 years to sharing and developing the teachings of Paramhansa Yogananda. Walters is author of more than 70 books on spirituality, yoga, and meditation, and the founder of the Ananda World Brotherhood Communities throughout the world.

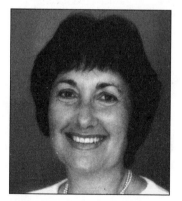

Devi Novak, the editor of this book, is co-spiritual director of Ananda worldwide and serves as an editor of *Clarity* magazine. She travels and lectures extensively throughout the world on the topic of emerging spiritual trends.

THE HINDU WAY OF AWAKENING:
ITS REVELATION, ITS SYMBOLS
An Essential View of Religion
By Swami Kriyananda (J. Donald Walters)
Trade Paperback, 349 pages

"...provides an understanding of Hinduism as the inner Way that all souls tread, characterized by profound wisdom and devotion, and with a genuine tolerance and appreciation of religious diversity that is so much needed in our world."
—*Light of Consciousness*

This book gives hope—for each one of us, for life, for the future. It is, as the subtitle claims, an essential view of religion; it points to that essence of eternal truth that animates every great religion in the world. *The Hindu Way of Awakening* reveals the vital connections between Hindu understanding and our modern life and culture. The author provides keys to understanding true soul awakening beyond mere identifications as Hindu, Jew, Christian, etc. *The Hindu Way of Awakening* views Hinduism not as a popular religion of ceremonies, exotic religious images and allegories, but as Sanatan Dharma, the Eternal Religion. Topics include revelation, symbolism, the Avatara, Brahma, Vishnu, Shiva, Tantra and the Divine Mother.

THE PATH
One Man's Quest on the Only Path There Is
By J. Donald Walters (Swami Kriyananda)
Trade Paperback, 420 pages with photographs

The Path is the fascinating story of one man's search for truth and happiness—bringing him to the door of one of the spiritual giants of this century, Paramhansa Yogananda. Filled with insightful stories and mystical adventures, it gives the reader hundreds of stories of Yogananda, and an intimate glimpse into what it was like to live with one of the great yoga masters of modern times.

ART AS A HIDDEN MESSAGE
A Guide to Self-Realization
By J. Donald Walters
Trade Paperback, 189 pages

"J. Donald Walters has provided a manual for creativity as spiritual practice. Insightful, inspiring and imaginative, it reveals the sacred dimensions of artistic expression and opens a new world of meaning and purpose."
> —Michael Toms, co-author of
> *True Work: The Sacred Dimension of Earning a Living*

In *Art as a Hidden Message,* Walters reflects upon the moral, spiritual and human values of art which express life's true purpose and meaning. Art, music, and writing allow us to transcend ourselves, lead us to Self-realization, and inspire us to lofty thoughts and aspirations. This book offers a blueprint for the future of art, and shows how art can be a powerful influence for meaningful existence and positive attitudes in society. Here is a new approach to the arts, one that views both artistic expression and artistic appreciation as creative communication. Walters shows the importance of seeing oneself and all things as aspects of a greater reality, of seeking to enter into conscious attunement with that reality, and of seeing all things as channels for the expression of that reality.

SECRETS OF MEDITATION
By J. Donald Walters
Gift Paperback, Color photographs, 68 pages

Finalist—Best New Age Book, 1998 Ben Franklin Award

"The secret of meditation is unifying your inner and outer life: offering every problem up for resolution to the peace within; allowing that peace to infuse your outward activities."
> —*Day Twenty-Nine*

Full of inspiring, helpful tips on meditation, this little desktop guide offers a seed thought for every day of the month. It has been said that we are what we eat. It would be truer to say, "We are what we think." For our minds express, and also influence, the reality of what we are far more than our bodies do. *Secrets of Meditation* is a potent guide to meditation that points the way to the deeper levels of inner peace that we all seek. The book contains 31 daily affirmations to help you bring the essentials of meditation into your life. Beautiful color photographs accompany each affirmation.

THE ESSENCE OF SELF-REALIZATION
The Wisdom of Paramhansa Yogananda
Edited by Kriyananda (J. Donald Walters)
Hardcover, Trade Paperback, 211 pages

"A wonderful book! To find a previously unknown message from Yogananda now is an extraordinary spiritual gift."
— *Body, Mind, Spirit* magazine

The scope of this book is vast—it offers as complete an explanation of life's true purpose, and the way to achieve that purpose, as may be found anywhere. A few of the chapters include: The True Purpose of Life; On Meditation; How to Pray Effectively; The Law of Karma; The Lesson of Reincarnation; and Ways in Which God Can Be Worshiped.

AUTOBIOGRAPHY OF A YOGI
By Paramhansa Yogananda
Reprint of the Philosophical Library 1946 First Edition
Hardcover, Trade Paperback, 481 pages with photographs

"...an eyewitness recountal of the extraordinary lives and powers of modern Hindu saints, the book has importance both timely and timeless."
— W.Y. Evans-Wentz, M.A., D.Litt., D.Sc., Jesus College, Oxford; Author of *The Tibetan Book of the Dead*

"In the original edition, coming from the period of Yogananda's life, one is more in contact with Yogananda himself. It is prior to his institutionalization that often follows many great personalities once they have passed on. ...While Yogananda founded centers and organizations, his concern was more with guiding individuals to direct communion with Divinity rather than with promoting any one church as opposed to another. This spirit is easier to grasp in the original edition of this great spiritual and yogic classic."
— David Frawley, Director, American Institute of Vedic Studies

Followers of many religious traditions have come to recognize this book as a masterpiece of spiritual literature. Yogananda was the first yoga master of India whose mission it was to live and teach in the West. His first-hand account of his life experiences includes childhood revelations, stories of his visits to saints and masters in India, and long-secret teachings of Self-realization that he made available to the Western reader. This is a verbatim reprinting of the original 1946 edition of *Autobiography of a Yogi,* with all its inherent power, just as the great master of yoga first presented it.

THE RUBAIYAT OF OMAR KHAYYAM EXPLAINED

By Paramhansa Yogananda ♦ Edited by J. Donald Walters
Hardcover, 354 pages

"The most enchanting reading experience I've had in a decade."
—Wayne Dyer, Author of *Real Magic and Everyday Wisdom*

Nearly 50 years ago, Yogananda discovered a scripture previously unknown to the world. It was hidden in the beautiful, sensual imagery of the beloved poem, *The Rubaiyat of Omar Khayyam.* His commentary reveals the profound spiritual mystery behind this world-famous love poem, showing the deep allegory of the soul's romance with God.

MEDITATION FOR STARTERS

By J. Donald Walters
Trade Paperback, 135 pages

Finalist—Best New Age Book, 1997 Ben Franklin Award

"A gentle guide to entering the most majestic, fulfilling dimensions of consciousness. J. Donald Walters is a wise teacher whose words convey love and compassion. Read and listen and allow your life to change."
—Larry Dossey, M.D., author of *Prayer Is Good Medicine*

"Gives both beginning and longtime meditators proven techniques and powerful visualizations to heighten contemplative experiences. Highly recommended."
—PJ Birosik, *New Age Music News & Reviews*

Meditation brings balance into our lives, providing an oasis of profound rest and renewal. Doctors are even prescribing it for a variety of stress-related diseases. This award-winning book offers simple but powerful guidelines for attaining inner peace. Learn to prepare the body and mind for meditation, special breathing techniques, ways to focus and "let go," develop superconscious awareness, sharpen your willpower, and increase intuition and calmness. *Meditation for Starters* is available as a book & CD set, book & cassette set, and as a 79 minute video. Each item is also sold separately.

Companion CD or cassette: Includes further instruction on meditation. In the first 30 minutes, learn the fundamentals of meditation plus step-by-step instruction. The second half contains a beautiful and deeply interiorizing visualization set to soothing music, entitled Land of Mystery.

Companion Video: This 79 minute video is divided into two parts. Part I includes a talk and instruction by Walters, interwoven with an enchanting guided visualization set to music. Part II is the entire *Land of Mystery* visualization without instruction.
J. Donald Walters is one of the leading authorities on meditation and yoga in the world today.

ANANDA YOGA™ FOR HIGHER AWARENESS
By Swami Kriyananda (J. Donald Walters)
Trade Paperback, Lay-flat binding, 160 pages with photographs

This handy reference book covers the basic principles of hatha yoga including standing poses, relaxation poses, spinal stretches, and inverted and sitting poses, all with photographs. Includes suggestions for routines of varying lengths for beginning to advanced study. Swami Kriyananda is the founder of the Ananda Yoga for Higher Awareness system. Kriyananda was often asked to demonstrate yoga postures for his guru, Paramhansa Yogananda, (author of Autobiography of a Yogi) in the late 1940s.

AUTOBIOGRAPHY OF A YOGI ◆ AUDIO BOOK

By Paramhansa Yogananda ◆ Read by J. Donald Walters (Swami Kriyananda),

6 cassettes, selected chapters, approximately 10 hours

"Kriyananda has a voice that enthralls, and a vision that ennobles."
—Haridas Chaudhuri, author and philosopher

This audio book is taken from the verbatim original 1946 edition by Paramhansa Yogananda. It includes the key chapters of *Autobiography of a Yogi,* read by Swami Kriyananda, a close, direct disciple who lived and studied with Yogananda. Listen to an individual who has dedicated the past 50 years of his life to living and sharing the teachings of Paramhansa Yogananda. Kriyananda's gentle voice and deep understanding of Yogananda's words are a delight for listeners wanting to experience this spiritual classic.

THE RUBAIYAT OF OMAR KHAYYAM EXPLAINED ◆ AUDIO BOOK

By Paramhansa Yogananda ◆ Read by J. Donald Walters
Includes the 75 poetic quatrains translated into English by Edward FitzGerald
4 cassettes, 96 min. ea., total: 6 hrs., 27 min.

Enjoy some of the most evocative and spiritually insightful verses ever written. Yogananda's allegorical explanations of Khayyam's famous poem will awaken listeners to the deep spiritual truths behind this literary classic. Listen to the melodic voice of J. Donald Walters as he sings each verse, reads the poetic paraphrase, then follows with a clarifying, expanded meaning.

KRIYANANDA CHANTS YOGANANDA

by Kriyananda (Donald Walters) ◆ vocal chanting,
approximately 70 minutes, CD/cassette

A direct disciple of Paramhansa Yogananda, Kriyananda chants
the spiritualized songs of his guru in a unique and deeply inward
way. Throughout the ages, chanting has been a means to achieve
deeper meditation: let this music uplift your spirit.

MANTRA

by Kriyananda (Donald Walters) ◆ vocal chanting, 70 minutes,
CD/cassette

For millennia, the Gayatri Mantra and the Mahamrityunjaya
Mantra have echoed down the banks of the holy river Ganges.
Chanted in Sanskrit by Kriyananda to a rich tamboura accom-
paniment.

"Ancient, unhurried majesty." —NAPRA Review

THE MYSTIC HARP

by Derek Bell ◆ instrumental, 70 minutes, CD/cassette

Original melodies by Donald Walters capture the mystical quality of traditional Celtic music. Derek plays Celtic harp on each
of the nineteen richly orchestrated melodies and is joined on the
title New Dawn by noted violinist Alasdair Fraser.

*". . . an ambiance quiet and dreamy enough to appeal to new age
audiences and Celtic folkies."* —*Billboard* magazine

"Utterly radiant, with noble simplicity and innocence."
—NAPRA Review

MYSTIC HARP 2

by Derek Bell ◆ instrumental, 72 minutes, CD/cassette

Derek Bell is the harpist for the five time Grammy award winning
Celtic group, *The Chieftains.* In this sequel to our best selling Celtic
album, *The Mystic Harp,* Derek displays his legendary artistry in over
twenty new original melodies written by Donald Walters.

To order or to request a free catalog, please call:

Crystal Clarity, Publishers
and Clarity Sound & Light

800-424-1055 or 530-478-7600
Fax: 530-478-7610

E-mail: clarity@crystalclarity.com
or visit our website:
www.crystalclarity.com